Ivan Vaughan

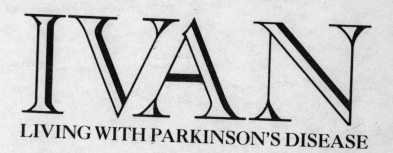

IVAN
LIVING WITH PARKINSON'S DISEASE

With an introduction by
Jonathan Miller

PAPERMAC

Note to the Reader
**Changes in medical treatment for a condition
such as Parkinson's disease should be made
only after discussion with a doctor.**

First published 1986 by
MACMILLAN LONDON LIMITED

First published in paperback 1988 by
PAPERMAC
a division of Macmillan Publishers Limited
4 Little Essex Street London WC2R 3LF
and Basingstoke

Associated companies in Auckland, Delhi, Dublin, Gaborone, Hamburg, Harare,
Hong Kong, Johannesburg, Kuala Lumpur, Lagos, Manzini, Melbourne, Mexico
City, Nairobi, New York, Singapore and Tokyo

British Library Cataloguing in Publication Data
Vaughan, Ivan
 Ivan.
 1. Parkinsonism —— Patients —— Biography
 I. Title
 362.1′96833′00924   RC382

ISBN 0-333-46407-9

Printed in Hong Kong

Contents

Part Three

Dedication

David Marsden
Niall Quinn

Jan
Justin
Sophie
Paul and Linda
Jonathan Miller
Staff of Homerton College
Jon Alpert
Iain Wilkinson
William Langston
Mum
Bern
Birgit Kitchin
Patrick Uden
Anne and John Mulcahy
Charles Bailey
Gillie
Mimi
Britannia Pharmaceuticals
Merck, Sharpe and Dohme
Rita Cola
BBC Radio 3
Ruth and Arthur
Rick and Wendy
M. Csikszentmihalyi

A special acknowledgement is due to Stephen Platt
for taking on the role of amanuensis and
providing invaluable editorial assistance.

Acknowledgements

Scharlie Platt
Suzanne Glass
Katie Falcon
Karina Thistlethwaite
Sue Proctor
John Maltby and Vivien
MSC
REMAP
Crossroads
Cambridge City Council
A charity in the West Country
Brenda Stephenson
Nick Chapman
Roger Jefcoate
The numerous thinkers and research workers
who have influenced the development of my views
about Parkinson's disease.

Introduction

In 1817 the English physician James Parkinson described a disease of the nervous system in which the patient was progressively afflicted by a stooped, shuffling rigidity accompanied by a coarse disabling tremor of the limbs. Although Parkinson referred to this condition as a 'shaking palsy', it is not really a paralysis in the obvious sense of the term, because although the patient's movements are slowed, sometimes to the point of statuesque immobility, it is possible to overcome the rigidity and under the right circumstances the patient may surprise onlookers by moving with unexpected speed and fluency.

Viewers of the BBC documentary on Ivan Vaughan found it hard to reconcile the apparently normal running sequence at the start of the film with the strenuously awkward ritual of dressing in the morning. In order to make this transition, Ivan had to tumble off the front steps of the house and it was only by taking advantage of this self-inflicted emergency that he was then able to jog for several miles. And even then a trivial interruption, such as an unexpected encounter with a dog or a friend, could easily bring him to a standstill, at which point the trembling rigidity reclaimed him once again. The disorder displays many paradoxes of this sort. And as one clinician wrote in 1895, 'Parkinson's disease remains so utterly inexplicable that we are constantly drawn to it by the lure of the mysterious'.

The last eighty years have seen remarkable progress in neurological research, and Parkinson's disease is not quite as inexplicable as it once seemed. For instance, although there is still some dispute over whether the various examples represent one disease or several, the fact that so many of them are associated with degenerative changes in the same part of the brain – in the so-called *substantia nigra* – has convinced most neurologists that Parkinson's disease is, after all, a pathological entity.

Even so, the precise cause of the condition is still obscure and, although an important advance was made when it was discovered that the affected region of the brain is conspicuously deficient in the neuro-transmitter dopamine and that startling remissions could often be brought about by administering L-dopa, a metabolic precursor of dopamine, the treatment remains to all intents and purposes symptomatic and the improvement is not necessarily maintained when the drug is administered over a long period of time. Besides, it is notoriously difficult to stabilise the dose and, unless the progress is frequently monitored, the patient can easily exchange one set of disabling symptoms for another. The limbs may now be affected by slow twisting movements and, although these can usually be corrected by reducing the dose, some patients claim that even when it is working favourably the drug tends to induce a disturbing sense of coercion. So while Ivan Vaughan would be the last to deny the blessing of L-dopa, he would be the first to insist that the blessing is a mixed one, and that there is an enigmatic sense in which he is more 'himself' when he is off the drug than when he is relieved of symptoms and on it.

For that reason, and also perhaps because he is an unusually curious patient who regards his condition as something to be explored as well as endured, Ivan juggles with his own treatment and, in the knowledge that he can always run to the drug for shelter, he sometimes takes pharmacological holidays so that he can experiment with the transitions from one state to the next.

As far as the medical profession is concerned, this sort of therapeutic improvisation is short-sighted and irresponsible, and any adjustments are best left to those who are in the know. But for an intelligently introspective patient such as Ivan Vaughan, having the disease is just another way of *being* in the know – and since the paradoxical experiences of the disease are quite literally unknowable to anyone except the sufferer, Ivan feels that he has valuable contributions to make and that the experiments are not simply frivolous self-indulgences.

The problem is that, although doctors pay lip-service to the principle that all patients should be listened to, the intelligent sufferer often comes away from the clinic with the distinct impression that he or she has been seen without actually being heard. And since many of the vicissitudes of the disease cannot be observed and have to be described, the patient's spoken testimony is one of the most valuable sources of information.

Unfortunately, it is only too easy for the busy clinician to confuse a garrulous patient with one who is helpfully eloquent, and when it comes to someone like Ivan Vaughan, who sees himself as a partner in the research as opposed to being a submissive patient, professional hackles are raised and there is an understandable, but not altogether forgivable, tendency to close ranks and disparage such contributions as the ramblings of an eccentric amateur.

In that respect Ivan is undoubtedly an awkward customer, and it is not difficult to sympathise with the suspicion that he arouses – not only amongst neurologists but also amongst the members of the Parkinson's Disease Society, who prefer to maintain a co-operative relationship with the profession and feel that Ivan Vaughan's individualistic experiments rock the boat unhelpfully. All the same, as medicine becomes more scientific, its official literature leaves less and less room for the subjective accounts provided by the patient, and as the discourse becomes denser and more impenetrable, it becomes harder and harder to hear the voices of those for whom the benefits are designed. It is only by dint of his heretical awkwardness that Ivan Vaughan has succeeded in making at least one of those voices audible, and although both doctors and other Parkinsonian sufferers have argued and will continue to argue that Ivan's case is atypical and that his film appearance was both misleading and alarming, I feel now, as I felt when I reluctantly accepted his original invitation to visit him, that Ivan has a certain wisdom to impart and that anyone who is interested in this perplexing disorder has something to learn from him.

I can still remember my own irritation on hearing the thin, importunate voice at the other end of the telephone when Ivan rang me out of the blue with the request that I should come up to Cambridge and hear what he, a sufferer from Parkinson's disease, had to say about it. What, I thought, made *him* so special? Why did *he* rather than anyone else deserve a visit? To my shame, I tried to put him off, pleading business, not to mention a lack of requisite qualifications. But fortunately he refused to take no for an answer, insisting that I could surely spare an hour or two and that it was precisely because I was *not* a member of the neurological establishment that I might perhaps hear details that had gone unheeded by the better qualified.

It became apparent immediately on my arrival in Cambridge that my irritable misgivings were ill-founded. Ivan and I spoke for many hours and I soon became aware of the fact that, in some altogether mysterious way, he had succeeded in surmounting his disease by regarding it as a treasured possession and not just as an abominable affliction. As far as he was concerned, Parkinson's disease was simply another mode of existence filled with intriguing paradoxes, the introspective study of which might perhaps lead to a better understanding of the nature of normal will and action. After discussing the possibility of collaborating on a book, it was finally agreed that the subject might be broached more successfully in the medium of film – and from the awed fascination shown by the crew, I was convinced that my own interest was not peculiar and that what Ivan had to say and show would intrigue and enlighten the ordinary viewer.

The book in which Ivan now develops these themes will probably arouse just as many objections as the film did. His description of what it is like to suffer Parkinson's disease is unarguably idiosyncratic and no doubt fellow sufferers will claim that their experience does not square with his. And neurologists will probably take exception to Ivan's unremittingly combative attitude to the treatment that is now on offer. All the same, this controversial narrative provides an indispensable supplement to the 'official' history of Parkinson's disease. As Carlo Ginzburg says in the introduction to *The Cheese and the Worms*, historians who might once have been accused of wanting to know only about the 'great deeds of kings' are now turning towards what their predecessors passed over in silence, discarded or simply ignored: namely, the personal experience of anonymous people whose lives are often omitted from official descriptions of a particular period. Apart from the fact that Ivan's account has an undeniable value for its intelligence and for its inquisitive curiosity, and because extended subjective descriptions of this disease are so rare, its heretical tone of voice is just one of the things that future historians will find intriguing.

The amateur theologian rediscovered by Ginzburg represents the voice of an ordinary person who finds himself in conflict with the official dogmas of the Catholic Church and is prepared to risk and lose his life in the effort to reconcile his own beliefs with the teachings of the Vatican. By retrieving this story, Ginzburg has amplified and enriched our picture of moral and intellectual life at the end of the sixteenth century. I'm convinced that the future will recognise Ivan's contribution in the same light and that his argumentative heresies, which could so easily have been passed over in silence, will eventually be seen as a valuable document in the history of medicine.

Dr Jonathan Miller
May 1986

Part One

Diagnosis

'What do you think it is?' I asked a friend who was a doctor. He took hold of my left hand and we both watched and waited.

'There it is!' I said.

'It's hard to say,' he replied, 'but I think you should go to your own doctor and ask him to arrange for you to see a specialist.'

'Have you really no idea at all?'

'Well, it could be Parkinson's disease – but there are so many different types. I wouldn't worry about it.'

A few days later I went to see my GP. He gave me a stark choice.

'Either you can wait for three months on the National Health or you can be seen in a couple of days privately.'

Private medicine was against my principles, so I didn't like to have to make such a decision; but I had to make up my mind immediately and, unwilling to wait, I chose the earlier date.

It was a beautiful, hot day in June 1977 and, as I wanted the exercise, I rode the couple of miles to the specialist's house on my heavy butcher's bike. When I arrived I was sweating lightly. I sat down and answered his questions as accurately as I could while my thoughts rushed ahead, trying to make sense of what was being asked. I blurted out all the ideas I had about what was happening to me. Quietly, the specialist made careful notes. After a while he asked me to strip off. I lay on the couch and wondered what was going on as he began knocking my knee-caps and bending my arms.

'They seem all right.'

Then he took hold of my left hand. My little finger was jerking rhythmically.

'I think I'm a bit cold,' I said. 'Could you close the window?'

'Of course.'

When I was dressed again, I sat down and said casually: 'I hope it's not Parkinson's. But you must be honest with me and not hold anything back.'

I had no idea what Parkinson's disease entailed and I was hoping that, if that's what it was, it would prove to be an insignificant problem that could be overcome without difficulty. So I was jolted when the specialist said in a quiet, serious tone that, sadly, in his opinion, I did have Parkinson's.

I tried to remain casual and got up to leave, remembering the Marx brothers' joke: 'I've got Parkinson's disease, and he's got mine.'

The specialist looked surprised: 'I'd like to see you again,' he said, and promised to arrange an appointment for a couple of weeks' time at the outpatients' clinic at Addenbrook's Hospital neurology department, in Cambridge, where I live.

I had not asked him any details about the illness and I enjoyed the ride back. But once I was at home with my wife, Jan, I found myself saying: 'I'm very sorry, but I've got Parkinson's disease. Don't worry though, I'll get over it.'

Neither of us really knew what was involved. The uncertainty left Jan very disturbed and frightened, while I remained casually dismissive, determined to enjoy the challenge, convinced that I would meet it through will-power. Until I had cured myself, however, no one else was to know.

I felt I had a choice: I could either hand over the management of my illness to the experts, or I could keep control of it myself. I preferred the second approach. The illness was mine and I would make it my project: a journey of exploration. However, depending on how well I got on with the doctors, there was a third option of a continuing dialogue between myself and the experts in deciding what to do.

During my first visit to the hospital it quickly became clear that the time available to discuss ideas with Dr Iain Wilkinson, the specialist in the neurology department, was limited to one fifteen-minute session every six months. I had already spent hours preparing for the meeting and had loads of questions. I managed to blurt out only a few of the most important ones and I respected Dr Wilkinson for his honest replies.

'What's thought to be the cause?'

'I'm afraid we just don't know.'

'How quickly does it get worse?'

'I'm afraid we don't know that either.'

'What exactly is supposed to have gone wrong?'

'Well, there is an area in the brain called the *substantia nigra* . . .'

For some years I had been interested in the working of the brain and had tried to keep abreast of current knowledge. Six months earlier the BBC's Reith Lectures had been on 'The Mechanics of the Mind' and I had listened intently, just able to grasp the main points. I had brushed up my knowledge for the hospital appointment and was able to use and understand words like 'transmitter', 'neuron', 'synapse' and 'structural or functional damage'. I thought that if I showed that I was familiar with the jargon, I would be able to support my claim to retain control of the illness. I don't think Ian Wilkinson was fooled, however. His manner was warm and straightforward and he tactfully ignored the shallowness of my understanding. Even if my knowledge had been greater, though, there seemed to be an almost total absence of hard fact concerning Parkinson's disease.

As I passed through the doorway on my way out at the end of the interview a host of unasked questions began to crowd into my mind. I hadn't shown him the bump on the back of my head, or mentioned that my little fingers would not stay straight when I stretched my hands open. Both these idiosyncrasies had been commented on when I was a child. Could the bang on my head have disrupted the connections between brain cells and motor functions?

I had read that Parkinson's disease sometimes results from syphilis after a long period of incubation: what about that woman in Paris twenty years ago?

Could I have breathed poisonous chemicals from the extractor fans in the roof of the chemistry laboratories opposite my home? Maybe I had been poisoned by smoke from the load of firewood injected against Dutch elm disease that I had bought last winter, or by the traces of fertiliser in the bags the wood had been stored in?

What about dietary factors? In my usual mad way I had drunk six pints of milk a day on a holiday in France in an attempt to put on weight and, despite feeling drowsy and uncomfortable, had persevered in doing so for a couple of weeks.

Was there anything in the idea that a virus might be responsible? I had read a newspaper article on the amazing ability of 'flu viruses to survive. There had, of course, been the famous 'flu epidemic that swept the world in 1918, bringing in its wake a strange sleeping sickness that affected millions of people and left some of them with symptoms of Parkinson's disease – as Oliver Sacks describes so brilliantly in his fascinating book *Awakenings*. Perhaps that same virus still lay dormant and could reappear under appropriate conditions. Could it have been lurking beneath the keys of the old piano we had bought recently, waiting to be blasted into activity by my attempts to play?

Could it have been brought on by my weightlifting? Was it too absurd to suppose that I had caused the death of countless brain cells by trying to impress the instructor so much that I pushed myself in the exercises until

I got dizzy and almost blacked out? Could the pressure of the heavy bar on my neck have broken some nerve path between the brain and the spinal cord?

As a student I had lived in a room with a gas fire and gas ring but no ventilation. There had been no charge for the gas, so I used it excessively. Had spending long periods in an atmosphere depleted in oxygen caused brain damage?

Then there was the strange way that, during the last couple of years, my trouser belt tended to shift to the left so that the buckle was off centre. Was that loss of symmetry a sign of a gradual collapse of the left side of my body?

All these ideas crowded into my mind as I made my way home. What had really caused the disease?

Catastrophe

The cold December air flowed in under the blankets as, reluctantly, I sat up. My mind retained a drowsy sense of happiness from the joy and fulfilment of love-making, but my body felt like lead. The film of moisture on my skin had magically dried by the time I reached my clothes. I was due at the squash court at five o'clock. I dashed downstairs and slumped into the freezing car. After a few moments of uncertainty it started and I drove off. The heat from my body misted up the windows and I had to switch on the fan. As I parked near the squash courts of the college where I lecture in the psychology of education, I noticed that I was beginning to sweat slightly.

My friend and colleague Malcolm was hovering around the changing rooms waiting for me. I began to look forward to the game. We went up to the balcony to watch the previous pair and, as I sat there waiting for them to finish, I wondered if I had handicapped myself by making love. Perhaps the feeling of weakness in my legs would go once I started playing. This was usually the best time of the day for me to play. In fact, I'd been interested to see that other players seemed to avoid early afternoon bookings, even if all the morning ones had been filled, but were quite happy with the four o'clock to six o'clock slots.

As soon as the court was free we went in and slammed the door shut. As if in another world, I let myself go completely, rushing about in all directions, whooping and shouting, smashing the ball against the walls. I loved the sense of freedom.

A racket was spun and it gave Malcolm the serve. It was a classic battle between my speed and his accuracy. Speed won the first game. I was boiling hot and took off my T-shirt; Malcolm was still wearing his track suit. The match was the first to three games. My aim was to leap, dash and slam my way to victory as quickly as possible. The score passed through seven–five in my favour, then he pulled back to seven–six. Two long rallies took it to eight–seven to me, and gave me the serve. It was a good one and the ball tippled down into the corner, but Malcolm slammed it against the back wall and the ball sprang forward, went in and limply dropped to the floor. There was assessment and decision in the incredible lurch I made. Having reached the ball in time, I flicked it to the right. I'd won the second game.

I didn't like asking for a couple of minutes' break, but I needed to recover. My chest, neck and face were bright red. My skin felt clammy and I lay stretched out, heating up the wooden-block floor. Malcolm had now taken off his track-suit pants but, to my surprise, kept the top on. He won the next game easily. I was beginning to recover, but Malcolm had hardly warmed up. My game was weak and awkward and the score was nine–one to Malcolm. In the fourth game I made him run a bit more, but when the score reached seven–three, I decided to conserve my energy for the final game.

Malcolm took off his track-suit jacket but did not seem to be sweating or even hot. I was already preparing myself for defeat. After all, the reason for playing was for the pleasure of physical exertion rather than for victory: the process was more important than the product. Somehow that thought helped me improve my game. I went for the more difficult shots. I was ahead at three–two. Then Malcolm won the next point by delicately placing the ball way beyond my reach and my performance collapsed – first into helplessness, where my efforts failed to match Malcolm's returned standard of play, then into hopelessness, where I was incapable of making any effort at all. I did not score another point. We played a couple of friendly games before I would admit to myself that I was finished. I loved this feeling of exhaustion, followed by a warm shower. Malcolm calmly put on his track suit. He did not need a shower; in fact he had not even bothered to bring a towel.

As I left my skin felt damp, and by the time I had reached the car a cold sweat bathed my body. The car would not start straight away, so I sat back hoping the battery would recover its charge. I couldn't see a thing through the steamed-up windows. I rubbed the rear-view mirror with my fingers and could see the droplets of sweat on my forehead. Eventually the car started and I drove home quickly, went straight to the bathroom, rubbed myself down and climbed into bed. I set my mental alarm for an hour later, but woke after only twenty minutes. My hair was practically dry and I felt alert and energetic. I decided to go to the gymnasium after all.

I always felt excited as I approached the building, particularly if any of the windows were open. The clanking of iron broke into the quiet of the cul-de-sac outside. Once inside the building I walked quickly down the corridor to the changing room and was soon greeting Jeff, a fellow club member, who was lying back on a bench resting after a series of difficult lifts with weights far beyond my own capability.

I had been trying to fit in a session at the gym for a few weeks and, having finally made it, I was keen to get into weightlifting again quickly. To avoid criticism from Jeff, I kept to the appropriate weights at first. He did his best to guide me and keep me on a sensible curve of progression from lighter to heavier; however, I was impatient and, whenever I pushed myself to lift a higher load, I quickly adopted that as the new standard. After quarter of an hour he had gone and I slid additional weights along the bar and locked them in position. Aping the professionals, I gave a loud shout on the 'snatch' as I pulled the bar from chest level up to a position above my head before dropping it down with a mighty clang. I tended to hold my breath: it seemed to help produce the extra strength I needed.

There was a routine of different activities. I went over to the bench fixed into the wall-bars. You hooked your feet into straps and stretched out backwards with your head down towards the floor. Then with your hands behind your head, with or without weights, you curled up and tried to touch your knees with your forehead. I started with the bench at an angle of forty-five degrees but had to accept a shallower incline. A few weeks ago I had been able to do the forty-five degree bench, but now I was very much out of practice. I forced myself to stay for another half-hour in spite of the boredom that always seemed to replace my initial surge of enthusiasm when I exercised indoors. I missed out the lift where you set up a bar with weights between two stands at shoulder height and then position yourself so that the bar is resting on your neck and your arms are bent: I did not want to risk doing this exercise when no one was around to take the weights if I found myself unable to locate the stands for myself. I had got into difficulties doing it a couple of months before and had felt a strange sensation in my neck afterwards.

Like Malcolm, Jeff never seemed to sweat. He did not mind the heat, and had asked if I would mind not opening the windows. Now he had gone, I opened all three wide. Soon I was sitting in a current of delicious cold air, leaning forward, elbows resting on a bench and flexing my arms with a variety of weights. Circuit training was no good. I wanted to build my muscles as well as strengthen them, to have all the features of my person functioning in the fullest and richest way possible. Accordingly, the meal I ate when I arrived home was huge. It was not scientifically worked out, but every bit of it tasted delicious.

My friend and fellow lecturer John Ahier phoned and invited me over to his home in Wilbraham, just outside Cambridge, for a drink. I did not feel like going out again, but it had been quite a while since we last got together to criticise college and generally pull people apart, so I decided to go. A log fire and soothing lighting set the scene for my Cointreau and his whisky. We moved backwards and forwards between scouring academic board papers for controversial college policy, reviewing the way we marked essays and discussing friends and their relationships. We were chagrined to think of our artist friend Phil's likely success with his paintings. John brought me up to date with life in his village. I had sold my old Renault for thirty pounds to a village lad who thought he knew a lot about cars; John had seen it abandoned on a lonely stretch of road in the middle of the Fen and we debated whether I should give him his money back. We watched the late-night movie. Besides the whisky and Cointreau there was John's home-made sloe gin to enjoy.

Strong coffee helped to restore my confidence about getting home and at about three-thirty I set off, singing aloud bits and pieces of songs. The stretch of road between Cherry Hinton and Cambridge was often patrolled by the police, and I was right to worry about it. I checked and rechecked my speed but I was followed all the same. I was very nervous and my foot was shuddering slightly on the pedal.

The police car stayed with me as I drove into Cambridge and over the Hills Road bridge and turned down Bateman Street. There was no doubt that they were following me. My indicators flashed profusely at every turn I made. Down Panton Street. I wondered if I could make it home, with that sharp turn left and then an immediate turn right into the drive to the back entrance to the house. I held off using my indicator till the last moment and, as I made the left turn, I saw the police headlights signalling to me. I ignored them and swung round into the drive. I switched the engine off and sat there. Would they believe that I had not seen their signal, that they had left it too late? Would they convince themselves they could not win them all? Or would they come marching up to my car and breathalyse me?

I was terrified and for what seemed an age did not dare move in case they were out there listening for the click of my car door. Eventually I carefully squeezed the handle and got out. Everywhere was quiet. They must have gone on.

I crept into the house and noticed how late it was: it had gone four o'clock. I got undressed, apart from my T-shirt, in the kitchen and tackled the stairs. A couple of creaks would be sufficient to wake Jan, but it would be obvious that I was trying. I ignored the bathroom and the promptings of my bladder. Painstakingly I entered the spare bedroom and at long last reached the bed. There were no blankets, just a sheet, and it was freezing cold. As I stood there wondering what to do, I felt an unusual glow of warmth which gave me the impression that it was getting warmer and that the sheet would be adequate.

When I had got into bed, I was amazed at how wide awake I felt. After what must have been half an hour I thought, 'This is ridiculous, I must get some sleep.' I had a huge erection. I lay awake a bit longer. I was reluctant to masturbate myself to sleep, but I had a nine o'clock seminar and I was never going to drop off in that state.

'Oh, what the hell!' When the deadpan moment of excitement had passed, I adjusted my position and waited for sleep. I was feeling hotter and hotter and beginning to sweat. I was more awake than ever. I could hardly believe it. I wafted the sheet to let in the cold air. It did not seem to have any effect. There I lay, awake and increasingly alert. My sexual readiness kept repeating itself, despite numerous attempts to exhaust it. Despair took over. I searched for a dry section of the sheet and lay for a long time continually sinking towards sleep, only to be prodded back to wakefulness by the panic of being out of control that seized my brain. I was shivering. I was ready now to go for some blankets and face the consequences of disturbing the household, but the effort of raising myself was too great. I could neither make my limbs move nor even conjure the idea of getting up. Co-ordination would not come automatically and it was too great a burden to think through the necessary sequence of movements.

I don't know whether I fell asleep or not before the light filtered through the curtains telling me that it must be about eight o'clock. Once I had managed to get to my feet, I felt all right – maybe I was someone who needed very little sleep – and made it on time to the seminar I had to teach. Because I felt I ought to be showing the effects of the previous night, I looked among the students for signs of boredom or irritation, but could detect none. As I went about other tasks during the day, however, I suspected that I was less efficient than usual: things that should be done together or in sequence had to be done in separate bits.

It was not until bedtime that I got the first hint of something unusual going on in my brain. I turned to Jan and told her of a weird sensation in the back of my head – a throbbing, bopping sound as if the inside of my brain were twitching. As I climbed into bed I said casually, 'Perhaps I've had a stroke.'

The following summer my Parkinson's was diagnosed.

A Statement of Intent

'Hi, Ive. How did it go?'

'Oh, Iain Wilkinson's a lovely bloke, Jan; he's dead straight. So little time, though.'

'What did he say about the drugs?'

'He was very good about that. We discussed L-dopa. He said he was convinced I'd feel better on it, but he wouldn't put me under any pressure because he respected my determination to cope without drugs.'

I noticed a flicker of disappointment in Jan. I had a deep-seated aversion, which I had inherited from my mother, towards taking drugs and I had never even taken an aspirin. It was an attitude closely linked to my need to feel personal control over my emotions and what I did. It also fitted in with one of my main ideas about the disease: if I'd got myself into this situation it was going to be me that got myself out of it.

Jan's view was quite different. She was much more ready to accept the notion that we are helpless in the face of infections and diseases. She thought that in most cases they were unavoidable and it was just bad luck if you were the one to get caught. If you were ill you were daft not to take whatever medication was available. She did not have much time for notions of 'mind over matter', neither in the sense of psychological factors being responsible for the illness appearing in the first place nor in the sense of sheer will-power being the main factor in achieving a cure.

The guiding principle of my life, which I have held since childhood, is one of openness to novel experience. At times this means unreserved intellectual curiosity: open-mindedness, impartiality and a constant refusal to be dogmatic. At other times it is not a matter of intellect so much as an eagerness for experience and an unreserved pragmatism with a hedonistic content.

No commitment is sacrosanct; yet while I espouse an idea, it is held with total conviction. I have always resolved the paradox by claiming that my commitment is tentative. Jan is puzzled by and frequently objects to the way in which I can fervently hold one view over a long period of time and then suddenly switch and become committed to a totally different position. I argue that sometimes the evidence reaches such a level that a change is warranted. I have always revelled in my ability to take on complexity and to accept the contradiction and lack of consistency in many of my actions and attitudes, feeling that, as long as I do not try to convert people, and provided that the interests of others are not prejudiced by what I do, then there can be no objection to this idiosyncratic philosophy of life.

Both Jan and I knew that my hard-line position against taking medication would eventually be replaced by a willingness to accept it. However, the vehemence of my stance made her worry that it might be a very long time before I changed my mind.

The trouble was that Jan was highly implicated in the consequences of any decision I made concerning the illness. I denied this to myself for a long time and exaggerated the degree to which I was succeeding in maintaining my independence for coping from day-to-day.

As well as this self-deception, I was absolutely determined to conceal from friends and colleagues that I was ill and, when I could no longer keep it secret, to minimise the seriousness of the illness.

I felt as though I were standing in front of a dam. The walls were springing leaks in different places one after another. I raced round frantically trying to patch them up, but with my eyes closed in case I caught sight of the flood of water that threatened to engulf me. I could not acknowledge the seriousness of the illness because if I did so fear and panic would undermine the self-confidence I was still able to generate.

'Can't you see, Jan – it's a race between my developing ways of coping and people finding out about the illness. I accept that I've got the illness, honest, but I've got to pretend that it is not too serious, otherwise I'll be too intimidated to deal with it.'

'Look, Ive, it's your illness. Whatever I say or think, it is for you to decide what you want to do and I'll go along with it as best I can.'

How could it be true? I didn't get ill. Anyway, I was young and fit and only old people got Parkinson's. It was cold comfort that it was pretty extraordinary to get the disease at my age and that at least it supported my desire to be different and unique.

My father, who was a policeman, had been killed in the war when I was two years old. My mother had trained as a shorthand-typist before she got married and, despite the war and police pensions she received for my father, she had to go out to work to provide for me and my two sisters. When I was five she got a job as a school dinner lady so that she could be at home when we came out of school, but when we were older she took a job as a clerk-typist.

My mother had strong ideas about not being dependent on others, and she instilled this into us when we were very young. Throughout my time at primary school I had opportunities to develop my self-reliance and this tended to separate me from other children of my age. For example, I was able to handle relatively large sums of money to buy my own clothes – even costly items like macs and jackets. I used to take great pride in getting the tram into town and going into a shoe shop on my own, seeing the surprise on the face of the shop assistant as I tried on different styles.

A continuous conflict bubbled away inside me: between, on the one hand, wanting the security which comes through being the same as other children and, on the other, seeking to extend my individuality. Not having a father emphasised my difference, and neighbours played a crucial role in enabling me to build on this by establishing him as something of a legend. There was a story, which I never had any reason to question, about my father swimming across the Mersey (which for years I thought was the same as swimming the Channel). There were other tales of his exploits and physical prowess. He'd travelled round the world as crew on sailing ships, and whenever his name was mentioned in conversation it was accompanied by an aura of admiration.

With this picture of my father, and with my mother encouraging me to be independent, I grew up feeling that I could somehow make myself. Friends might have served as a model with which to identify, but I soon found that they could be unreliable. I have never forgotten my friend Nigel ramming his three-wheeler bike into the gate of my house after we had quarrelled and calmly saying, 'I'll be your friend, but I'm glad your father's dead.' So I sought to keep the influence of others at arm's length until I had laid foundations for myself that were sufficiently stable to provide me with a source of inner confidence and security.

After putting so much effort into developing my character, I was not going to climb down from my stance against taking the drugs. Parkinson's disease, I'd been told, was progressive and irreversible. I would show that it was possible to confound this prognosis and that the illness could be manipulated to serve my own ends. I didn't know whether I had the full-blown illness or whether it might take years to progress; or, even if I had got it badly, whether I would have the will-power and fitness to resist it or control it so that it wouldn't dominate or distort my outlook on life.

While using my physical strength to keep the disease at bay, I would use my intellect to research it. I would use myself as a test-bed to conduct an intensive case-study on my own pattern of response to the progress of the illness. I would find out all I could from the available literature and make contact with specialists in the field, who, I was sure, would leap at the chance to join me in this unique, in-depth case-study. At this stage I really believed I as going to make a breakthrough. I was capable of making it for myself and of having a good time in the intellectual exploration. I would keep away from others who were going to give in to the disease.

Stress and Security

Severe illness brings into sharp focus the choice between acceptance and resistance. My desire for independent self-determination pursued without compromise is based on the experience that, come the crunch, the customary forms of stability and security – parents, family, friends, religion – had all proved fallible. Childhood friends had moved on; they had become famous and I had been forced to cut my emotional ties with them. New friendships did not run as deep.

Intellectually I have always rejected too close an emotional contact with other people which could leave me susceptible to accepting their ideas. I pride myself on my ability to resist peer-group pressure, to stand back and appraise the 'facts'. In the heat of an emotional exchange with another person, ideas are more difficult to resist. I need time to reflect, without social pressure. That was my attitude even at school, where I refused to use the notes given out by history and geography teachers, preferring to go straight to the textbooks instead. I reasoned at the time that if the material had been accepted for publication it was less likely to be a biased, partial view.

I had abandoned religion when my childhood notions of a Father Christmas type of Christianity dashed against rationality. When the tremor broke out and I tried to calm myself to retain control, old mantras from childhood came flooding back, but I had to reject them. There was an ingrained refusal in me to fall back on non-rational props.

Yet in some ways this refusal to acknowledge emotional pressures is paradoxical. Despite my strong preference for wanting to take ideas from books rather than from live interchange, I read very little fiction and enjoy social relations. I have a fear of uncertainty but, having experienced it so much, I am able to cope with it and in some circumstances seek it out, even manufacturing high levels of risk. In the past this has resulted in a frequent switching between rational reflection and temporary bouts of elation in which I was on self-induced 'speed' and craved the stress. In this mood I could haul myself out of a morass of introspection, analytic precision, compulsive checking and pedantic qualification, my self-generated excitement allowing me to trip lightly and creatively over intricate problems.

Throughout childhood I used to whip myself into states of euphoria as the class clown, or by inducing excitement through stress – for example, by stealing money. Once I opened a drawer in the teacher's desk containing a box full of two-shilling pieces that had been collected for a school trip. I took the money over a period of a week, thinking that if the amount went down bit by bit no one would notice. Each night I crawled excitedly under my bed to watch the pile of coins growing steadily higher. On the Friday, the teacher announced that the money had been taken and asked whoever had done it to see him.

A wave of terror passed through me and by the following Monday I could stand it no longer. I went home at lunchtime, brought back all the money and persuaded the boy who had been left in charge of the remaining funds to let me look after it while he went out to play. As soon as he had gone I pulled open the drawer and carefully emptied my pockets into the box. They would not all fit in, so I put the surplus in loose. Then I left. Two days passed and still nobody noticed that the money had been returned. The following day I volunteered for dinner-time guard duty. After waiting five minutes, I opened the drawer and, even though nobody was looking, gave a big shout and rushed out of the classroom and down the corridor to the staff-room: 'Sir, the money's back!'

I blurted out the story of how I had thought to check if the remains of the fund were still there and had found that all the money had been returned. 'Amazing,' said Mr Holmes, and the matter was pursued no further.

This was not an isolated incident in my childhood and adolescence. Looking back, it seems almost as if my life was an apprenticeship in stress and the art of coping. I sought pressure as a means of inducing a high. At the time I realised dimly that I was being driven into activity rather than choosing action, and now I wonder whether I was compelled by a desperate longing to find a theory to cope with hereditary and social limitations. Attempts to rationalise personality result from a driving need to generate the resources of hope and energy necessary for survival. Having practised these strategies repeatedly throughout my childhood, I had learnt to harness resources for coping with day-to-day emergencies, so prior to the appearance of my illness I was tuned to a very high pitch in dealing with self-induced stress.

John Lennon

'I'll telephone John.'

Although both John and Paul had helped me financially in the past, this was not what I needed now. I believed that to exist was to be in the minds of others, and the higher your regard for the person who was thinking of you, the stronger your awareness of your own existence. John had lived in New York for years and contact between us had been sparse. I was deeply moved whenever he made a friendly gesture towards me. In my present turmoil I was prepared to induce such a gesture by letting him know about my illness.

After a lot of rummaging I found his telephone number, but it was two years old and people in his position frequently change their numbers. However, it was worth a try. I remembered to take account of the time difference, sat next to the telephone and dialled. Nothing. No tone, no voice, no indication of why I had not got through. I looked again at the figures scribbled in my diary. Was it 262 or 212 for New York? This time I'd try 212. There was a ringing tone and then John's unmistakable voice: 'Yeh?'

I automatically dropped into a Liverpool accent. ''ello John. This is Ivan, 'ow a' ya doin'?'

'Just a minute. 'ow do I know you're Ivan? What did you have painted on your tea-chest?'

' "Jive with Ive, the ace on the bass." '

'OK. I 'ave to do that 'cos people keep gettin' your name from books about the Beatles and ring up pretendin' to be you. So 'ow are you? 'ow's Jan?'

'She's well. 'ow's Yoko and Sean?'

'They're beautiful.'

We talked for a while, and I felt pleased that he took the time to clear up false impressions that I might have gathered about him from the press. Then, in the middle of the conversation, I let out that I had Parkinson's disease. He had heard of it and volunteered to get me some books to help. I was as impressed as ever by the warmth he could generate in just a few words, and by his sharp intuition when he said, 'You'll have more time to devote to the things that really interest you, like archaeology.' Before we spoke, I had been thinking that I would be able to read more about travel and archaeology.

Putting the phone down, I went to the sitting room and sat down. I was amazed when I realised that it had been three years since I last spoke to him. I had nothing special to do and sat there all afternoon thinking about him and our childhood together. How extraordinary it is that attitudes and values laid down in early life permeate the adult personality whatever the experiences in between.

I met John when I was three or four years old. One wet morning there was a knock at the front door. My mother opened it, and looking down, found a boy a bit older than me, smiling, but preoccupied with the effort of remembering what he had been rehearsed to say.

'I believe a little boy lives here. I wondered if he might like to come out and play.' He stood there in the porch, rain pouring down behind him, with a pair of slippers under his arm.

'Come on in. What's your name? You live round the corner don't you?'

Next day I went round to the house where he lived with his aunt and uncle. We played with Dinky cars. I was surprised by his generosity and willingness to share his toys; he was happy even for me to take some of them home. When his Uncle George came home with some sweets John readily shared them. There was an immediate bond between us. He was older, read books, and his greater intelligence and experience were apparent. I accepted his leadership but I was determined to preserve my independence. From the warm security of Aunt Mimi's control, John accepted me into his life.

John was a member of his local library and immersed himself in books so that by the age of five he was already a fluent reader. I was still in the infants' school when he started at Dovedale Road Primary School, but we played together after school and at weekends. There were numerous parks, a golf course, and fields full of tangled growth and trees – just right for playing cowboys and indians. In one barren area with large lumps of hard earth we played football and cricket. We spent hours digging out tracks to race our Dinky cars. Our most exciting game, though, was 'fires'. We would go to a large area of waste ground and simply set fire to the straw and watch the blaze. I have never understood why nobody stopped us.

John's gang comprised, besides himself, Pete Shotten, Nigel Walley and me. I was the youngest and was constantly having to prove my worth. I felt privileged to be John's friend since he was nearly two years older. He protected me against Jimmy Tarbuck and his gang on the rare occasions when I made the mistake of confronting one of them.

John and I went to different grammar schools, but I used to hear about the chaos and riot that seemed to be a daily feature of his schooling. I rather lost touch with him when I went to university, and did not see him again until some time after I was married. Then one day, as I was playing with my little boy Jus on the steps of our house in London, a white Rolls-Royce turned into the road. John jumped out followed by a woman I had not met before.

'Hello, Ivy! This is Yoko.'

'Yoko who made the bottoms' film?'

'Yeh, have you seen it?'

Jan and I had been to see it by accident a few months before. We had stayed for three-quarters of it and I had found it genuinely original.

We sat round my kitchen table. John took a biro, drew a diagram and said: 'This is what Apple's all about.'

The word Apple appeared in the centre with various divisions, including records, shop, electronics, films and foundation, radiating out.

'This is where you come in,' he said, pointing to the word 'foundation'. 'I want you to set up a school.'

Trying to keep calm, I asked him to explain what he had in mind. He hadn't thought beyond the broad idea of a school embracing the most child-centred of regimes which his children and those of his friends could attend. The timing was right: I was just finishing some research, so I said yes.

Arrangements were made to incorporate me into the structure of Apple and I began to formulate plans. My priority was to come up with a scheme for a school which was not simply for children of rich parents. Meetings were arranged, the outline of a steering committee established and numerous properties visited.

Apple's accountant argued that the school was not a viable proposition, since the required funds were simply not available. Paul McCartney, whom I had known well since the third year of secondary school, did not share John's blind faith in the project. Feeling discouraged, I made contingency plans. I had to be careful to prevent disappointment turning into depression. When taking on extravagant goals I had to justify the value of any lesser achievement. In the end it all came to nothing, but I persuaded myself that it had been worthwhile. I had made numerous contacts and there was the possibility that one day the project would be revived.

My attachment to both John and Paul ran deep and occasionally I would go to great lengths in order to see them at a moment's notice. Maybe Paul saw our continuing friendship as a way of maintaining simple values he held dear. Jan liked Paul, though she did not see much of John. She was not the least bit mesmerised by their fame. She enjoyed eating at expensive restaurants and sampling London's nightlife, into which Paul took us from time to time. But, should the effort become too great, she was willing to let the relationship fade.

A month after telephoning John in New York, a heavy parcel was delivered. It was not until I was reading the titles of the books it contained that I realised they had been sent by John and Yoko. There was one by Arthur Janov, author of *The Primal Scream*, and one entitled *Mind Magic*. *How to Get Well* had on the fly-leaf a message from John that read 'to start looking', and *The Snow Leopard* had a note saying 'to relax'. This last book gave me the greatest pleasure and I frequently re-read passages from it. Its author, Peter Matthiesen, lost his son through illness and journeyed in Nepal and Inner Dolpo on a completely pointless journey to catch sight of a snow leopard. The peace that he found travels across to the reader from each page.

John's accompanying letter urged me, in punning language, to keep my spirits high and strongly suggested that it was up to me whether I sank or swam. I must not lose faith in myself.

Ten weeks later he was shot dead. Paul and I did not contact each other about it; in fact, we never brought it up in conversation. I hardly reacted outwardly at all. The day after John's death, however, a colleague said that he supposed I was very upset at what had happened. I heard myself say: 'I don't know what I feel. I don't know that I feel much at all.'

As soon as he had gone, I instinctively made my way to a room where I knew I could be alone, and I wept profusely.

Keeping It Secret

During the first few months, keeping the illness secret from other people was fairly easy. I could not stand the thought of having to put up with people feeling sorry for me. The last thing I wanted was to be regarded as 'in-valid': I wanted to go on being seen as a person to be reckoned with. I did not want to fall into the position where allowances or excuses had to be made because of difficulties of one kind or another.

At first it was simply a matter of clenching my left fist in order to squeeze the tremor out of my little finger. I was curious to know where the tremor went – if it went anywhere at all. I soon noticed that it became worse the more emotionally aroused I was. Interestingly, the tremor broke out whether I was distressed by something unpleasant or excited by something enjoyable. In the calm that followed a period of arousal, the tremor often disappeared without the need to squeeze.

In college, I noticed that some people were becoming aware of the strain I was under while others remained completely ignorant. The ploys for disguising the tremor became increasingly elaborate as the symptoms began to involve more muscles. I began by sitting on my hands and in the common room would seek out chairs that had sides to hold on to. During whole conversations I would sit with my arms folded and my fingers straining to maintain a grip on the hollows of my rib cage. At other times I could be seen standing with fingers intertwined, hands clasped behind my head, my bent arms flapping backwards and forwards in harmony with the flow of the conversation like a nervous stork about to take flight.

The policy of not telling anybody gradually proved more and more difficult. If I kept in one position for more than a short time, a kind of rigidity began to set in. If a student stopped me in the corridor with a complex problem needing careful thought and attention, I used a kind of dance routine to try to cope with the arousal and consequent loss of control: I would clench my fists, put my hands behind my back, then behind my head, twining my fingers together, cross my arms and finally, when all else failed, I would lock my trembling arms behind my back.

I hadn't a clue what my facial expression was signalling at times like this. I suspect that over and above the general aspect of tension there would also appear moments of pure panic as my already divided attention completely lost contact with the conversation in order to concentrate on maintaining control of my body. Above all, I had to avoid resting for too long in one of the coping postures and getting stuck.

Those who knew me well and were not completely blind began to notice changes in my manner and behaviour, and more and more people must have begun to revise their opinion of me from an easy-going and light-hearted to a serious and excitable person.

Even simple, straightforward requests could be an impossible trial. For example, someone might ask me for copies of journal articles I had promised to lend them. The terror that could flash across my face at being unexpectedly interrupted in what I happened to be doing would be misinterpreted and would set in motion a complex process of apology by the other person, accompanied by an urge to impress upon me that the articles were not needed urgently – in fact, not really needed at all and that they were sorry for bothering me. Inevitably this would be followed by my attempt, usually futile, to reassure them that it was no trouble and that the material was on my desk simply waiting to be collected. They would then offer to collect it themselves; I would counter by almost begging them to believe it was absolutely no bother. Finally, I would break away before the interchange spiralled into total absurdity.

I tried to avoid meeting people. I hid from friends I met in town and pretended I was not in when friends came round. Jan and I refused invitations to dinner parties or to visit friends. If I could not avoid seeing people, I would refrain from telling them what was wrong. I always preferred to be thought of as odd rather than as someone who was seriously ill.

My determination not to take drugs made life difficult for Jan. People were beginning to ask if there was something the matter with me. I took a hard line and Jan had to follow my instructions in saying that I was fine. She tried to show me how awkward she felt and suggested that other people's enquiries were well meaning. I said that if they wanted to indulge in idle speculation then that was their business: I wasn't going to satisfy their curiosity. She was silly to let such a trivial problem upset her. I was convinced that I was successfully disguising my illness. Jan was feeling increasingly uncomfortable as she sensed the kinds of interpretation that was being put on my behaviour. I insisted she was only imagining things. I professed not to care what people thought so long as they were unable to pigeon-hole me as disabled with all that that might imply.

Jan was right though. Much later, after I had made the announcement at work that I had Parkinson's, it became clear that people had thought I had become an alcoholic, was on drugs, was having a nervous breakdown, or that Jan and I were splitting up.

There was an interim stage between keeping it totally secret and letting everybody know. I selected four of the senior members of college to receive a copy of a letter I sent to my head of department, Charles, in which I set out the policy I wanted to pursue at work. I wrote: 'The more I am in a position where I have to accept that there is something wrong with me, the more I perceive a loss of control. This leads to feelings of inadequacy, which in turn lead to anxiety. This emotional arousal in turn exacerbates the symptoms.'

Trying to avoid this spiral of anxiety was a major motive in trying to keep the disease secret. As it became more and more difficult, I blamed Jan for not trying harder to help me dissimulate and for letting the difficulties depress her, which put further pressure on me. In the end, though, I was forced to recognise that the policy of secrecy and the problems it entailed imposed a whole new range of anxieties and a consequent exaggeration of the symptoms.

At college, Alison, the Principal, asked to see me. Having welcomed me into her room, she said she was sorry to hear my news. I replied that I'd been preparing myself for this sort of crisis all my life: I welcomed the challenge and would be able to cope. She offered to help in any way, taking great care not to offend my desire to uphold my position as a full member of college. She said she was sure colleagues would carry me. I thanked her, but later I was puzzled by what she had meant, since she also offered to give me an address for details about breakdown pensions . . .

Professor Marsden

I had always liked the idea of being someone who stood out, and I had cultivated the difference between me and my more conventional colleagues. I liked to think I was less constrained in my relations with students. Now, with my illness, I set about developing compensatory activities to maintain my status. I invited Colin Blakemore, an eminent neuro-physiologist and an expert in the field of perception, to talk to the philosophy discussion group I belonged to.

'How are you, Ivan?' Colin asked when he arrived.

'Terrific, thanks. How are you?'

'Very well.'

'In fact, I'm not that good,' I blurted out. 'I've got Parkinson's disease.'

'Oh really? Are you sure? Let's talk about it after the meeting.'

The philosophy group met informally three times each term in college to discuss a broad range of issues, mainly of relevance to education but occasionally focusing on more general topics. I enjoyed these talks and the careful analytical nature of the debate. I also enjoyed the cut and thrust and scoring points. Feelings of reward could, however, prove a Pyrrhic victory if the opponent had been weak, because one always risked getting trounced later by stiffer opposition.

I was fascinated to see how far attitudes expressed reflected general personality and values. I'd noticed the way in which some speakers would stubbornly hold on to their position when counter-arguments appeared totally convincing. Their public stance was allowed to change only in private. After a suitable time had elapsed, the opposite argument might be trotted out for all the world as if they had worked it out for themselves. Clearly, in spite of extensive training, professional philosophers found it as difficult as everyone else to avoid commitment to a particular viewpoint and to ignore the emotion that accompanies public debate.

How far an individual could be objective and rational was for ever humming away at the back of my mind. There seemed to be an important question concerning the bias arising from an individual's mood at the time of adopting an idea. In the same sort of way as memory is coded to particular emotional states, so the key to objectivity might involve the individual in spinning through a whole range of emotional states to obtain as many different slants to an idea as possible – but this seemed rather far fetched unless one used drugs to warp oneself through as many different states as possible.

The greater the personal contribution to developing an idea, the greater the commitment and attachment to it. This attachment becomes an addiction when there is high emotional involvement. When the ideas impinge on security or physical well-being – for example in severe illness – then it is much more difficult to risk abandoning beliefs because so much more is at stake.

A philosopher might claim that the procedures for practising his art are sufficient. I thought that, although people shared a common language to conceptualise their experience and ideas about the world, nevertheless ideas are biased by emotions. Each person builds his own model to interpret reality and achieve greater understanding. My concept of openness and rationality must also be socially conditioned. Objectivity is a matter of degree.

After the meeting, Colin told me that he was a good friend of Professor David Marsden, one of the world's leading experts on Parkinson's disease and, if I liked, he would contact him on my behalf. My hesitation must have been apparent, because Colin added that it was perfectly in order for it to be arranged within the National Health Service.

The journey to London to see Professor Marsden lasted two and a half hours. I took a taxi for the final stage to avoid being late. I had already had to cope with the anxiety of the trip, and for some reason taxis always make me very nervous. Their meters don't help: I become obsessed with the clicking increase in the fare, inexorably charging time, even when we aren't moving.

When I arrived at the Maudsley Hospital, where Professor Marsden worked, I had a long walk through a maze of corridors before coming to a broad lobby where I was able to tell a nurse who I was.

'Ah yes, would you like to come over here?' I moved to take off my coat and was surprised when she immediately stepped forward to help me. The implication of this for the progression of my illness unnerved me.

'No, it's all right, I can manage, thank you.' I was surprised, too, by her offer of a chair. Was I reading too much into these gestures of welcome, or was I right to conclude that patients with Parkinson's regularly needed such support? All I had was tremor in my hands and occasionally in my legs, but I could stand up all right.

She showed me into a cubicle. Soon a man walked in briskly and, without introducing himself, shook my hand.

'Come and lie down over here, will you?' He proceeded to carry out the same test on my reflexes that Iain Wilkinson had used. Like Iain, his manner was calming and considerate.

As I lay there I snatched a couple of glances at him.

'Can't be Professor Marsden. He's too young – he can't be more than thirty-five. He must be one of the Professor's assistants.'

He finished his examination and I followed him into a large room where about twenty or thirty white-coated students sat waiting.

He was very generous with his time, spending almost an hour describing the illness and giving me plenty of time to ask questions. I was quick to get into my stride and confidently told him my experiences so far, almost cockily illustrating the way I coped with any difficulties that arose. I told him I now had to make my lectures doubly interesting in order to hold the students' attention against the possible distraction of my tremors.

As the time passed and I was still waiting for Professor Marsden to appear, I began to think that, although his assistant was able to answer my questions with an air of authority and conviction, it was a pity that after such a long journey I would be unable to see the Professor himself to show myself off as an interesting case that would provide lots of ideas for discussion and, possibly, for research.

One of the main things I wanted to ask was whether I was doing myself any harm or accelerating the progress of the illness in some way by not taking the available drugs. I put this to the doctor and his answer was unequivocal: there was no evidence to suggest that I would be causing further damage by not taking the drugs.

'I can appreciate that you want to keep the powder dry for as long as possible,' he said.

I was now armed with ammunition against anyone who might persist in trying to make me take the drugs, with remarks such as: 'I realise I don't know anything about it, but it seems to me that if the drugs are available, you should take them', or 'It's none of my business, but I read somewhere that there are drugs which cure your illness.'

As I turned to leave, wondering if Professor Marsden might appear at the eleventh hour, the doctor stretched out his hand and said, 'Good luck.' I was momentarily stunned. Significance was piled up on top of these two words as I started to retrace the path up and out into the open air. What was I going to need luck for? Did his experience of Parkinson's disease suggest I was going to need a lot of it?

A week later I thanked Colin for helping to arrange the visit, but added that I was a little disappointed not to have seen Professor Marsden himself.

'I don't understand,' he said. 'I spoke with him the other day and he mentioned his session with you.'

My discomfort and embarrassment quickly gave way to pleasure that I *had* made contact after all.

Personal Enquiry

A month before my visit to London to see Professor Marsden I had tried to explain to Iain Wilkinson in a letter where my observations and thoughts seemed to be going. Some of these early ideas now seemed wide of the mark and somewhat fanciful. Nevertheless, it was a start – and I already knew that, provided I received the slightest bit of encouragement, I would never be able to sit back and hand over the illness to the experts. I wrote:

> I very much appreciate your straightforward approach to my problem and to my seeking to postpone treatment as long as possible. No doubt I shall seek treatment within the next few years, if not months. In the meantime, can I use you to receive a few notes which do not require a reply? It's simply for me to feel secure that what is happening is known by someone who can interpret it better than I can.
>
> It seems to me that a host of things are associated with the 'illness' in one way or another, including body temperature, arousal, time of day, alcohol, sleep. I can't be sure it is connected, but concentrated alcohol, such as whisky, seems to be associated with some change in blood pressure in the night, which is accompanied by tension and numbness of certain limbs. I can't judge whether numbness is a bad thing or not. I'm assuming that if it's allowed to last, there's a greater risk of muscle deterioration or a take-over bid by 'emotion' for the control mechanisms. It's as if the threshold of control for the left hand, and arm, has been breached and there is little chance of recovering that. But the rest is still controllable in so far as, under normal circumstances, I can force the 'emotion' to move elsewhere.
>
> However, I'm not sure about the usefulness, other than as a delaying tactic, of exercise. If my right hand is loaded with tension and emotion, I can reduce it through exercising the hand and arm. For the first time the other day I lost total control when it came to writing some notes. The attached bit of paper shows the hopeless effort at 4 p.m. and its improvement following some wrist exercises an hour later. I

would like more guidance on the most appropriate kind of exercise. The bottom end of my back seems to ache easily too. But, of course, all this may be due to distributing the tension when I seek to control the left hand. I'll ring you about it.

It's as if strenuous exercise breaks down muscle and leaves it open to erosion by 'emotion'. If it is moderate, it may strengthen the capacity to resist. Do you think, therefore, that moderate exercise may help, or at least do no harm in the sense of accelerating the processes leading to deterioration?

I may pursue the hypnotism angle I mentioned when I saw you. I talked with someone who thought it might be interesting and useful. I keep an open mind about it and will try not to go in for any of the more outlandish approaches. I've turned the whole thing into a game, a battle of my will over my primitive emotional centres!

It was very useful to be a member of the University Library. It had all the books and journals that anyone could want. I eagerly set about trying to fill in the huge gaps in my knowledge so that I could begin to understand and appreciate the significance of the research findings on Parkinson's disease. I felt I must protect my strong motivation from being undermined through the difficult jargon, statistical analyses and obscure concepts concerning brain functioning.

Each time I visited the library, particularly if the weather was warm and sunny, it was like entering an Egyptian pyramid. The porters at the entrance desk would inform you in too loud a voice if you misbehaved: 'Your card is out of date, sir', 'Not that staircase!', 'You are only allowed four books with a blue form'. I spent many happy hours searching the stacks for references, groping in the darkness when the time-switch for the lights ran out.

Early on I found a copy of James Parkinson's *Essay on the Shaking Palsy*, published in 1817. His description of the history of the disease was accurate and daunting:

> The first symptoms perceived are, a slight sense of weakness, with a proneness to trembling in some particular part; sometimes in the head, but most commonly in one of the hands and arms. . . . After a few more months the patient is found to be less strict than usual in preserving an upright posture: this being most observable whilst walking. . . .
>
> Hitherto the patient will have experienced but little inconvenience. . . . But as the disease proceeds, similar employments are accom-

plished with considerable difficulty, the hand failing to answer with exactness to the dictates of the will. Walking becomes a task which cannot be performed without considerable attention. . . .

At this period the patient experiences much inconvenience, which unhappily is found daily to increase . . . writing can now be hardly at all accomplished; and reading, from the tremulous motion, is accomplished with some difficulty. Whilst at meals the fork not being duly directed frequently fails to raise the morsel from the plate: which, when seized, is with much difficulty conveyed to the mouth. At this period the patient seldom experiences a suspension of the agitation of his limbs. . . . Harassed by this tormenting round, the patient has recourse to walking, a mode of exercise to which the sufferers from this malady are in general partial. . . .

But as the malady proceeds, even this temporary mitigation of suffering from the agitation of the limbs is denied. The propensity to lean forward becomes invincible, and the patient is thereby forced to step on the toes and fore part of the feet, whilst the upper part of the body is thrown so far forward as to render it difficult to avoid falling on the face . . . being, at the same time, irresistibly impelled to take much quicker and shorter steps, and thereby to adopt unwillingly a running pace. In some cases it is found necessary entirely to substitute running for walking. . . .

In this stage, the sleep becomes much disturbed. The tremulous motion of the limbs occur during sleep, and augment until they awaken the patient, and frequently with much agitation and alarm. The power of conveying the food to the mouth is at length so much impeded that he is obliged to consent to be fed by others. . . .

As the debility increases and the influence of the will over the muscles fades away, the tremulous agitation becomes more vehement. It now seldom leaves him for a moment. . . . The power of articulation is lost. The urine and faeces are passed involuntarily; and at the last, constant sleepiness, with slight delirium, and other marks of extreme exhaustion, announce the wished-for release.

I didn't like the recommended cure either:

. . . blood should first be taken from the upper part of the neck. . . . After which vesicatories should be applied to the same part, and a purulent discharge obtained by the appropriate use of the Sabine Liniment.

I was unable to restrict myself to papers on the behavioural aspects of the disease. I accepted that there were discrete specialisms for tackling a problem area like Parkinson's and felt that the really interesting findings were in biochemistry. My knowledge of chemistry was nil, yet it seemed important to ensure that a model at one level of description and explanation was consistent with detailed knowledge from other specialities. For example, if I hypothesised that the resources available for carrying out plans interact with and affect the ability to formulate a plan, then it seemed vital to check that at the neural and biochemical level there are pathways and modes of transmission that make this possible.

I soon discovered how vast the literature on Parkinson's had become. I would sit in the library flicking through the *Journal of Neurology*, skimming over the summary, introduction and the discussion at the end of the papers with no hope of understanding the major part in the middle. I owed a debt to Karl Pribram of Stanford University, whose books spanned the gap between psychology, human behaviour and neurophysiology.

I was bewildered by the labels: neuro-biology, neuro-physiology, psycho-physiology, psycho-neurology, psycho-pharmacology. This spawning of new specialisms revealed the extent to which the dialogue between different disciplines was already underway and how teams of specialists from each field were getting together to do research.

What all the references and reports seemed to agree on was that there was still no known cause of Parkinson's disease.

The symptoms characteristic of the disease – tremor, muscular stiffness and slowness of movement – had been recognised for over a hundred and fifty years. In Paris in 1915 a medical student named Tretiakoff showed that these symptoms reflected a dysfunction of a region of the brain called the *substantia nigra* – a deeply pigmented nerve-centre about the size of a large bean.

A major step forward came in the early 1950s when doctors in Sweden demonstrated that this collection of nerve cells produced and stored a chemical called 'dopamine'. They discovered that the nerve cells of the *substantia nigra* send long, thin fibres to connect with other nerve cells deep in the grey matter of the cerebral hemispheres. Dopamine was shown to travel to these cells to act as a chemical messenger transmitting nerve signals and it was proved that a deficiency of dopamine, owing to an injury to the *substantia nigra*, led to the symptoms of Parkinsonism. How that region of the brain becomes damaged remained a complete mystery. How frightening – a disease without a cause!

Another major breakthrough was made in Sweden in 1957, when Professor Carlsson suggested a metabolic precursor of dopamine, 'levodopa', might be used in the treatment of the disease. This led to research in medical centres throughout the world and ultimately in L-dopa (Levodopa) being formally approved for use in 1970.

L-dopa is now the standard treatment for Parkinson's disease. After all the exposure it has received on television and in the newspapers many people regard it as the wonder-drug that has 'cured' Parkinson's disease. The fact is, though, that it wouldn't cure the damage to my brain and although it would mask some of the symptoms, it would also produce other adverse effects.

From my reading, I realised that, although there was considerable research in progress, there were many questions still to be answered, leaving plenty of scope for someone like me to make a real contribution. It required an intellectual giant to be up to date in a variety of fields; Pribram struck me as one, and David Marsden seemed to be another – but I would see how far I could get on my own before I contacted him again.

Cycle Ride

It is 6 a.m. and I am wearing fingerless gloves, cycle clips to trap the air round my legs, and my Levi jacket with buttons to undo if I get too warm. It's my favourite kind of weather: a light breeze from the southwest. Skimming round the corner down Fen Causeway and over the mist-enveloped bridge, I pedal on, my muscles free to go in different directions instead of being pulled into taut rigidity. I play games as I ride, swinging my body backwards and forwards, whistling and humming with pleasure. It's chilly, but I'm warm and feeling fluent. I'm able to keep the balls of my feet in position on the pedals. I have the road to myself, unconcerned about the bike, not thinking what I'd do if something went wrong.

Cambridge is way behind me and fields stretch into the distance on either side. On the right the road passes over a new by-pass to leafy Coton, offering a short ride back to Cambridge; straight ahead is the longer route and I take that one. As I freewheel down the other side of the bridge, the relationship between effort and joy seems clear. There are three ingredients: the memory of having surmounted a difficulty; the additional pleasure that comes from an achievement of one's own making; and finally, at a physiological level, the feelings of elation induced by the abundant release of chemical resources in the brain to cope with the task.

With a spurt I catch up with the milk-float and pedal on to Barton. My bike is an ordinary one, with conventional handlebars and three-speed gears. There is a bit of play in the crank but it doesn't bother me. It's comfortable and I like its dark green colour and the original lettering just visible along one of the bars. Left down the Haslingfield Road and past Lord's Bridge Observatory. A disused rail track carries the huge white discs of the radio telescopes, finely tuned to eavesdrop on the stars.

It is still fairly cool but blueness is beginning to get the better of grey. The farmhouse in the distance comes into sight and I feel in my pocket to check that I've brought some money. I pedal a little faster as I approach the farm and the old wooden table standing in front of the pond. I climb off my bike, lean it against a tree and survey the home-made jam, tomatoes, cucumber, apples and eggs. I fill my bike-basket, put the money in the jar and continue: left through the silent corridor of trees and houses, and left again along the country route that begins the journey home. As I gaze over the distant fields I feel light-headed and at peace.

The steep slope of the bridge over the sunken by-pass comes into view; my mind responds and I decide to have a go. My muscles soak up more energy and respond with a brief burst of speed. More slowly now, breathing in a regular rhythm, feet squarely on the pedals, bottom lightly touching the saddle . . . I imagine a catapult as my attempt gains speed. Passing the base of the bridge, the powered momentum carries me halfway up. As the bike slows my body rises off the seat and, standing on the pedals, I press down on the writhing machine, zig-zagging a path up the last stretch until my front wheel lurches on to the flat top. With a final push I plonk back into the saddle and pedal easily across the bridge. I pull on the brakes and swing off the bike. The sun is now warm and everywhere is coloured by a strong light. The occasional lorry drones by beneath as I stare straight ahead, slowly munching an apple bought at the farm.

I remember train spotting on an autumn morning like this in childhood, swinging out of bed at daybreak and creeping from the house by the back door. It was cold; grey mist cut out the world. Once on the pavement a sense of release shot a sort of excitement through my body and I sat on the tram wide-eyed, shivering slightly in my pullover and short trousers as we moved away from houses, through fields of parkland and farms. The mist had lifted by the time I got to the railway bridge, but it was still cold and I tramped up and down to keep warm, waiting for the black shape to appear in the far distance.

After the huge blue engine had passed underneath, I took my pencil and a lolly stick I used as a ruler and, forcing my hands to stop trembling, drew the line that represented such an enormous achievement.

I sniffed and relaxed with the welcome smell of smoke in my nostrils. The next train was due in an hour and a half's time. I played games with myself to ward off the cold and pass the time. When daybreak eventually slashed the sky red, I felt a sudden glow of warmth which would stay with me all day. My love of the change from cold mist to warm clear sunshine had been laid . . .

A short burst from a siren interrupted my reverie. A police car raced away beneath me and my thoughts turned to getting home. I climbed on the bike and rattled down the steep incline from the top of the bridge. The air seemed to rush through a brain freed of anxiety and care.

Should I try to retain this peaceful state by committing myself to religious belief? Would I have to enter a state of mad euphoria to hold the disease at bay? Were compensatory resources released by spiritual ecstasy? I didn't want to relinquish the self that I had built up so carefully. When faced with difficulties, childhood conditioning sometimes prompted me to recite: 'The Lord is my shepherd; I shall not want. He maketh me to lie down in green pastures: he leadeth me beside the still waters.' That was all I could remember.

I wanted a notion of God that didn't rest upon myth. I was my own God. I was God, or, better still, God was part of me. The problem was to find the means to reach a state of godliness without being so completely bowled over as to forsake rationality. I couldn't accept dogmatic religious truth – a mixture of threats, promises, indoctrination, extraction of money, accumulation of property, idealisation of leader, the uncritical acceptance of written texts, the bigotry and intolerance. If one surveyed the whole range of religions and cults, they nearly all succumbed to these faults.

I sometimes found I could whoop myself up into such a state of emotional bliss that the symptoms of tremor momentarily disappeared. Had I simply mismanaged myself so badly that I had begun to sink and had forgotten how to swim? Had I transgressed a law of human nature proscribing self-examination by insisting on pursuing my enquiries? Had I severed a neural pathway by monitoring functions that should operate automatically to the extent that every move was executed with the brakes of self-regard jammed firmly in place?

I arrived at a narrow wooden bridge. I stopped by resting one foot against a post and traced the winding path of the stream along its tree-lined banks. I had to make a conscious effort to rest calmly in these surroundings, to hold back worries and pressing thoughts. Then a right turn for Trumpington and my legs pumped at the pedals to climb the long slope to the main road. Turning by the Botanic Garden, I realised I had allowed myself to waste the abundant flow in my brain that I would need for social confrontations that might arise later in the day.

I am home. It is eight o'clock. I'm fairly dry but I sit in a chair and quietly repeat nonsense to calm myself and avoid over-heating. Feeling good, I fill the kettle to make tea for Jan.

The Conference

A year after the tremor in my little finger first appeared I had to rethink my contribution to the college's in-service courses for teachers. To compensate for my reduced teaching efficiency I set about organising a massive conference on primary-school education. Henry Pluckrose, renowned throughout the world for his work as a primary-school head teacher in London, agreed to be the main speaker and I was fortunate to get two well-known politicians, the Conservative Rhodes Boyson and Joan Lestor from the Labour Party, to provide reactions to what Henry said.

I confidently managed the mass of correspondence and publicity, and an audience of three hundred booked to come. A couple of weeks before the conference, however, I began to doubt whether I would cope on the day. I remembered that during my meeting with Professor Marsden he had mentioned a drug which, although much less effective, did reduce some people's symptoms without the adverse reactions of L-dopa, the drug I was resisting taking. I had noted it down on a piece of paper but couldn't find it when I got home. Now, with the conference in view, I rang Iain Wilkinson and asked him if he knew what it might be. Iain named a drug; it sounded right and, as he assured me that it was completely safe, I asked if I might try it.

During the run up to the conference I tried out the drug. It calmed me down, made my face pallid and substituted a general blandness for the excitability that I normally exhibited. I took it with success before a lecture to check that it helped me keep the tremor under control while I was speaking to an audience but, just in case something went wrong on conference day, I asked a friend, Dave, if he would introduce the speakers and chair the question-and-answer session if the need arose.

It must have been difficult for Alison, the Principal, to resist involving herself more fully in the preparations, since I did not keep her informed or seek her advice. I wanted it to be my own success, not diluted amongst other people. That way I risked less damage to the college's reputation if, for example, the questioning got out of control. The issues were sufficiently controversial to attract the national press. Alison knew me, so when she asked if I would see her a couple of weeks before the conference I knew that her suggestions would be made to appear as minor frills which did not diminish any of my control. She asked if it would be all right for her to give a small lunch party for the speakers and anyone from college I would like to invite. I had brushed aside the question of lunch, thinking that I would get some sandwiches or go to a pub, but I accepted Alison's offer and also her gentle request that Charles and Ray, two of the more senior members of staff, should be consulted to see if they could offer any assistance I thought might be appropriate.

As I had hoped, Henry Pluckrose was excellent at the conference, mixing passionate declaration and illustration of what child-centred education entailed with clear argument concerning the theory underpinning his commitment. After coffee, Rhodes Boyson spoke, but Joan Lestor had still not arrived. When Rhodes Boyson had finished, I stepped to the microphone and was about to launch into my own summary and views when I suddenly felt my left foot begin to tremble. I gripped the lectern and stood staring out over the hundreds of heads, wondering whether I should let David take over as arranged . . . when the door to a committee room at the side of the platform squeaked open and Joan marched forward.

'I can't say how pleased I am to see you, Joan,' I said, amid laughter from the audience. The tremor had gone from my leg and I was able to last out the rest of the morning.

At lunch I lost control during the trifle. In a flash, Ray and Charles were beside me as if to shield me from embarrassing exposure to the rest of the company. It dawned on me how carefully they must have prepared for potential crises. Trying not to let anyone see, I swallowed another red pill. I couldn't avoid feeling ashamed. I had to take the blame for anything that went wrong. Perhaps sensing my feelings, Charles gave me a broad smile and said quietly, 'The conference has been a triumph, a real triumph.'

I put my hand in my back pocket to get a tissue to blow my nose and found the piece of paper on which I had written the name of the drug suggested by Professor Marsden. The drug that had seen me through the conference was not the one he had recommended!

A Family Row

'Professor Marsden supports me,' I said, ignoring part of what he had written.

I had been using the summer vacation desperately searching for any means other than drugs to resist the general decline into immobility. Jan had found it impossible to remain dispassionate about what she saw. Still persisting in holding out against the drugs, I minimised the havoc that I was causing.

'If Professor Marsden saw you now I'm sure he'd advise you to start.'

'If he did it would be because my state is worse than it need be.'

'Oh, you're blaming me again.'

'Yes, I am. For instance, when we go for walks and I'm doing quite well, perhaps it's unconscious, but you keep raising issues that are loaded with anxiety and it ruins my fluency.'

'Those walks are often the only time we get to discuss the house, things that need doing, and Jus and Soph's schooling. The rest of your time you completely devote to your illness. I can understand that. All I expect is some recognition of the difficulty in dealing with you. I bet nobody else would put up with you and your demands.'

'I don't demand anything. You can buzz off if you like and I'll manage on my own. You're no help at all. No, that's not true. You're very good on the practical side, but spiritually you're a disaster. You make it completely obvious that you don't go along with what I'm doing. I get no encouragement. You barely notice my success and exaggerate when things go wrong.'

Jan was in tears.

'It's true,' I continued. 'You're very good going with me to the pictures and things like that, but you won't adjust. You won't accept the changes that are needed – and there are not that many anyway. Justin and Sophie aren't affected at all.'

'You refuse to see it. They're bound to be affected.'

'No they're not. So long as I don't get fed up and depressed, as long as I show them that I can put up with the illness and continue to do most of the things I did before there's no need for them to be the least bit worried. It's you and your manner which gets them going. I need someone to love me, not just look after me.'

'I'll say it again. You go and find someone who will put up with you. You're living in the past. Husbands help their wives these days. I know you can't, but you don't accept that I'm doing two jobs completely on my own. My teaching and running the house takes up all my time. Surely you can understand that life isn't as much fun as it used to be. You sometimes spend the whole day sitting in your chair or falling around the house.'

'That's your look out. You're so miserable and don't make an effort. We never laugh any more. If John Ahier lived here I would be much better than I am. He's cheerful and wouldn't keep dragging me down like you do.'

'You can go, Ive. If you don't, I will. Then you can spend all the time you want with these people who are supposed to be so amazing.'

I did not want her to stay and live with the situation because she felt she had a duty to do so. She had to want to. Provided we were aware of it, a degree of distortion might be necessary in which the bad things were played down and the good things exaggerated. This would be all right, so long as we knew what we were doing.

Jan walked out of the room; she was crying again. I sat there for quite a while, staring ahead of me, wondering why I was so horrible. But at the time I believed that what I had said was true: I was on my own when it came to keeping my spirit alive. I struggled out of the chair and stumbled down the hall into the kitchen where Jan was slowly cleaning the pans that had accumulated in the sink.

'I do love you really, Jan.' I stood there in the doorway with a slight grin.

Turning her head she blurted through her tears, 'Don't say that. You don't mean it. You say the things you say and expect me to believe that you love me.'

'The main me does,' I reasoned. 'You must realise by now that at certain levels I think one lot of things which I don't believe for a minute at another level.'

'I think you're mad.'

'So do I.'

'I can't forget what you said.'

'I don't expect you to. Just understand that it is only a bit of me that says it.'

It was eighteen months after the first signs of my illness. I was still determined not to acknowledge the full extent of my disability. I tried to disturb as little as possible the everyday lives of those close to me as I clumped round the house or fell on to my bed, rigid for hours on end. Small achievements, such as reading the newspaper – sometimes the only thing I did in a whole day – were puffed out to support my belief that I was coping fine. Half the time I was having to be dressed and fed by Jan.

Ever since we'd been married Jan had had to put up with my occasionally letting out a volume of abuse followed later by a change of mood and a complete denial that I had meant it or that it should be taken seriously. I often asserted that I was above moods and then, when contradictory evidence was overwhelming, I would clarify what I meant by saying that I might have different moods but I could move them around and choose what mood I wanted to be in. The weakness of having a self that was shot through with contradictions was converted into a virtue under the protecting umbrella of my principle of openness. But now I was forced to consider the possibility that my behaviour resulted from a fundamental lack of security.

What did I want from Jan? I professed to be the ideal person to fall in love with because my values and attributes were so fluid and ready to incorporate those of another person. I could be happily married to a wide range of personalities because my values and self were so capable of revision and appreciation. Jan, I felt, was the exact opposite: she was stable, consistent, principled, honest and loyal – a perfect counter to me, and I loved her. But I was quite prepared to pull her apart for not being different. I didn't know what I needed from her. In some frames of mind she was everything that I wanted. She was providing all the necessary background support and was managing to avoid encroaching on my strong commitment to coping emotionally with the ravages of the illness. At other times I would cry out for support of a different kind. When my attempts to cope fell apart, I would expect full allowance to be made for my reduced capabilities and special consideration for my difficulties. I would accept and play the part of the helpless invalid yearning for 'tender loving care'. Ultimately, I didn't know what I wanted.

Deciding to Take the Drugs

I stood back and tried to sort out the different considerations. I was on the brink of retreating from my hard-line position against the drugs. Need it be a retreat? Could I turn it into a change of strategy?

It wasn't that I had ignored the impact of the illness on Jan, but I still claimed that the children were completely unaffected. I thought I had managed to protect Justin and Sophie, then aged thirteen and eleven, from any emotional disturbance about my condition. There had been no sudden shock. My attitude to the illness enabled them to adapt to each stage of progressive deterioration without any emotional trauma.

Although I hadn't been blind to the hard time Jan had been having, I must have been callous to disregard it, and thinking that the children had been able to ignore my condition as I fell all over the place might seem plain daft. But, I told myself, if they worried it was not because of seeing me in a poor physical state; it was because of Jan's refusal to take things lightly in the way I did. But I must stop setting her up. Why didn't I simply accept that the physical strain was the main reason for going on the drugs? Psychologically, I couldn't have been more cushioned. The practical support I had couldn't have been better. It was the spiritual encouragement that was weak.

Rubbish. No one else would have put up with the demands I made. But Jan's low spirits affected my condition. I could just about manage to keep my morale up in the face of muscular difficulties, but it was hard to prevent being undermined by her unwillingness or inability to keep cheerful. Basically she didn't go along with my policy of holding out against the drugs. She was pleasant enough when I was in a good state, but when things got bad you could almost hear her saying: 'There you are. You're not coping at all. You're in a hopeless state.' She hardly ever encouraged me when I asked her to acknowledge that it had been a good day, or a good walk, or a good film, because I had been trembling only slightly.

On the other hand, it was only because Jan was able to disguise her concern and successfully absorb the pain that I had been able to adopt this independent stance. I ignored the other main reason for giving in, which was that I was about to start my sabbatical year and knew full well that if I was in a bad state I was not going to be able to cope with visiting schools, talking to children, interviewing teachers and dealing with all the unexpected problems that would crop up while conducting experiments.

Anyway, I reasoned, taking the drugs would not really be giving in. It would, in fact – but I was going to convince myself that a different interpretation was possible. It was still me that could choose. But could you call it choice if it was made clear that you were going to be faced with subtle and increasing depression in people around you if you didn't decide that way? I could choose to ignore that if I wanted.

But could I really ignore it if I claimed to be open and aware? Maybe all that stuff about being open and rational was rubbish. I distorted the importance I gave to what I saw in order to suit a preference that I already held. No, that's not quite fair. What I do is hold out for giving the evidence a fair loading and then only when I've made the decision do I go back and retrospectively re-evaluate everything to suit.

What a load of nonsense. Who was the 'I' that assessed all this evidence so impartially? It was like imagining a group of people who didn't know what I felt or wanted, then these disinterested jurors made their impartial assessment. But who selected the jurors?

Openness is a relative idea. All I could do was to hope to be as open as possible without necessarily succeeding in an absolute sense. Maybe my special quality was being able to move in and out of various moods and get my different points of view that way. Whichever feeling left the strongest impression determined how I acted.

Jan was what she was; I couldn't expect her to change and become exactly what I wanted. Anyone else would probably have caved in ages ago. She could only do her best. But that was the point: openness is all about being able to change yourself as you go along.

Being given only one choice, being trapped or forced into taking the drugs was no choice at all. I was trapped by physical circumstance into having to go on to the drugs. But the trap was of my own making. It existed because I defined my situation in that way.

After months of soul-searching I began to reach a new accommodation with myself. Taking the drugs need not necessarily be a capitulation to the inevitable, a cession of control over my life to management and manipulation by drugs. I didn't have to hand myself over to a regime of drug-taking imposed by doctors. While accepting the necessity of the drugs, I could still create an opportunity for a whole new field of exploration and personal discovery by managing and studying my own pattern of drug use. And besides there was sex. That was another big reason for beginning drugs. The muscular difficulties were getting in the way of making love.

My aversion to the idea of taking L-dopa was not entirely subjective. People were always telling me there was a new miracle cure or asking why I did not just take the drugs available, but it was not that simple. L-dopa could have serious side-effects. Particularly worrying were physical writhing and psychological distortions. A standard reference pharmacopoeia contained the following warnings to doctors prescribing L-dopa:

All patients should be monitored carefully for the development of mental changes, depression with suicidal tendencies and other serious anti-social behaviour. Psychotic episodes, choreoaform, dystonic and other severe involuntary movements, muscle twitching, blepharospasm, paranoid ideation, cardiac irregularities, palpitations, nausea, vomiting, dizziness, gastro-intestinal bleeding, duodenal ulcers, hypertension, phlebitis, hot flushes, blurred vision, dilated pupils, urinary retention, bowel disorder, sweating, hair loss. . . .

The list was endless. I did not know what some of the terms meant, but clearly L-dopa was a very powerful drug. The book said the occurrence of many of these adverse reactions was rare, but the overall impression was very worrying. In comparison, my old aversion to taking aspirin sounded as harmless as popping an after-dinner mint.

But was my objection to taking the drugs based on the principle of retaining control and resisting any dependence upon exogenously derived chemicals, whether or not there were any adverse effects? Or was it based upon the unpleasantness of the adverse effects themselves? How would I react if all these unwanted effects were overcome by medical advances in new drugs? Did I really want a cure for this splendid and challenging illness anyway?

That was the real question: on what, exactly, was my stance against drug-taking based – on pragmatism or on principle? The question went to the core of my self-constructed being. Or was all this introspection just flannel to hide my basic reason – which was a fierce pride: a pride arising from my self-image?

Going on the Drugs

Before giving in and deciding to take L-dopa I thought I would make one last-ditch attempt to find out if some other measures were still possible. What about will-power or diet? Ideally I would find a food that provided the chemical my body lacked, or a drug that might stimulate or retard the functioning of the damaged system. I wanted to find anything other than the drugs which were direct substitutes for structural loss – the loss of the cells that manufacture dopamine in the brain.

Professor Marsden had given a talk on the radio in which he reluctantly mentioned evidence that smoking might inhibit the development of Parkinson's disease. I approached Iain Wilkinson and asked if I might try nicotine chewing gum as I had given up smoking some years back and did not want to start again. He could see no harm in my trying it. But the taste was dreadful and, as so often happened with my own experiments, I lacked the theoretical medical knowledge to sustain my efforts and help me resist giving up as soon as excuses presented themselves. Gum-chewing lasted two weeks.

My friend John Ahier took snuff in an attempt to retain vestiges of his aristocratic past. Discovering that snuff was tobacco, I thought it might be another way of ingesting nicotine without the risk of lung cancer. However, since it had no noticeable effect on my symptoms, I stopped taking it after a week. I could have tried chewing tobacco, but I don't think Jan would have stood for me squirting foul sticky juice around the house like some old sea-dog. Of course, spinach worked for Popeye and I tried it until I felt I was turning green.

Amphetamine enhances the functioning of neural pathways in the brain, so I approached Iain again to try to convince him to agree to my trying this commonly abused drug. It is known that amphetamine encourages the release of dopamine, the chemical I was short of. I wanted support for my idea that my difficulties were owing to a malfunction rather than to the destruction of part of the brain. I was surprised at the strict control over the issue of amphetamine. Each individual tablet had to be accounted for. At university, seventeen years before, my doctor had been quite willing to prescribe amphetamines to help me stop dropping off to sleep around four o'clock every afternoon. Now I discovered that medical journals of that time had contained numerous warnings that amphetamine could induce psychotic crises of the kind I had certainly experienced. I hadn't been worried – it had made me euphoric – but Jan, who, like me, was unaware of the power of amphetamines, had been puzzled by my changed state.

Iain agreed to prescribe amphetamines and I tried them for a week. There was some slight change in my symptoms, but I felt that somehow I was overtaxing my system. Besides, I didn't like my hair to be so greasy. There was only one thing for it: I had to start the wonder-drug, L-dopa.

The drugs, in the form of oval blue tablets scored across the middle to help break them in half, contained a hundred milligrams of L-dopa and ten milligrams of Carbidopa. They are taken orally, pass through the stomach, get absorbed into the bloodstream and pass into the brain. The barrier that protects the brain from unacceptable substances, including dopamine, allows L-dopa to pass. Once there, L-dopa is converted chemically to dopamine, the neural transmitter I lacked. Carbidopa is added to prevent an enzyme in the gut from destroying the L-dopa before it reaches the bloodstream.

Just over two years after the disease was diagnosed I started on a modest dose of half a tablet every couple of hours. Iain told me I could increase the amount to one tablet if I liked and asked me to let him know how I got on. I was torn between two hopes. I wanted the drugs to work so that I could carry on my research; at the same time I was half hoping they might fail so that I could prove I had some as yet undiscovered disease. Absurdly, I did not mind if the disease was incurable as long as it was unique and left intact my individuality. I had a bubbling confidence that I would discover a cure, or at least brilliant ways of coping, which would confound the experts. Perhaps by standing on my head long enough I might be able to flush out the blockage that led to my malfunctioning!

'I'm worse on the drug than off it!'

'Come on, you've only been on it four days. Iain said it might take a few days to establish itself.'

'Four days should be long enough.'

'Increase the dose then.'

'I might get those awful side-effects.'

'Yes you might, but you've got to give it a try. You've no choice if you're going to continue your research.'

I increased the dose to one and sometimes one and a half tablets every three hours, making sure that I came off the drug for a significant part of the day and never taking it at night. If there were going to be adverse reactions, I wanted to have a chance to dissipate them each day and avoid a cumulative build-up.

Jan had begun to resign herself to the possibility that the drugs might not work and had been careful to avoid making suggestions and getting involved, sensing the delicate handling required if I was to keep going. But after two days of taking the increased dosage, I appeared in the kitchen: 'Jan, they've worked! It's amazing, but look, I'm perfectly all right again.'

Part Two

Research Sabbatical

I had made arrangements to spend three days a week in a primary school a few miles outside Cambridge. I was investigating motivation in learning and wanted to study the use of rewards in classrooms to see if they reduced children's interest rather than increased their desire to do well. I also wanted to test different explanations of why such undermining of interest might occur. I had devised a series of simple experiments to conform with the demands of scientific procedure, although my preference was for watching and interviewing the children, and encouraging them to interact with me and their teacher. Some would be given rewards, some wouldn't; some would be offered them but not given them; and some would be given them without having been offered them.

The sessions went well; I was happy because I would be able to collect the data I needed. But as I observed the children, I began more and more frequently to turn to the back of my notebook to write down observations about what I was experiencing with L-dopa. The notes on Parkinson's reached the centre of the book before the notes on the children. I found my ideas about the disease demanded to be recorded. Links between the research with the children and reflections about my personality – notions of control, freedom of choice, effort, pleasure and the effects of the drugs on these and many more concepts – began to dominate my thoughts to the extent that I finally abandoned the research to devote myself to studying the disease.

One of the most interesting things was the way in which the control provided by the drugs seemed to go underground during the night and emerge the next morning, usually as early as four o'clock. It was as if the chemical were quietly in storage, to be called upon when I chose to do something that required it.

I came off the drugs for ten days or so. I wanted to discover which parts of me were affected by the change, and by coming off the drugs I would be able to experience them at first hand. I also wanted to keep up to date with the progress of the disease. I didn't want to mask the symptoms and then be shocked to discover that the disease had been inexorably worsening in secret.

There was also my personality and my preference for all-or-nothing extremes. If I'd got the disease, then I wanted to experience the full-blown range and intensity of symptoms. I wasn't disappointed! Coming off L-dopa for up to a week at a time left me completely immobile and hardly able to speak. I would spend all my time flat out on my bed and would have to be helped downstairs to be fed.

Sophie Feeding Me

Feeding someone else is a complex skill. Whenever she was around, Jan readily performed the task without complaining that the children should do their share. Occasionally, however, either because there was no one else to do it, or through a feeling of altruistic confidence, Sophie would have a go. As with any specialised technique, it is a good idea to practise the right way from the beginning rather than allow the wrong method to get a foothold. The trouble is that food varies in consistency, texture and taste, and these factors are complicated by how the person being fed is feeling – whether he is hungry or not, or whether he is finding it difficult to swallow.

On one memorable occasion when Jan was out, Sophie indicated she was keen to help but also eager to get off to see her friends. The first mouthful came too quickly, hit my closed lips and was immediately withdrawn halfway, a spoonful of cottage pie hovering above the void between plate and mouth. I was stuck, speechless, producing minute popping noises instead of words to try to attract Sophie's eye and get her to move the spoon over the plate. I attempted, but failed, to lock her attention on my eyes and focus carefully down to the spoon with an expression of anxiety, in the hope that she would realise what I wanted before any more of the beans and gravy splatted down into my lap.

She was busy looking at the newspaper. My legs were taut in readiness for the impact of each glob of food. With a gargantuan puff, I pulled back resources of energy from my legs and pumped them forward to my vocal muscles. Psyching myself up with a ritual of five pop-poppings of the lips, I managed to launch a loud whisper: 'Soph!'

She turned her head briefly, pushed the spoon forwards at me and got past my still opened lips. The stainless-steel spoon clunked against my precious uncapped front teeth.

'I thought you were telling me you were ready.' I gave a tight little jerk of my head to indicate that that wasn't what I had been trying to say, and stared down at my lap.

'Oh, sorry,' she said when she saw the splodges on my trousers. She put the spoon back on the plate and returned to her newspaper. My muscles were released from the agony of anticipating her dropping a whole spoonful on me and I was able to speak again.

'Soph, please concentrate. Get a kitchen towel and use the serving spoon.' I resolved, yet again, to make a special journey into town to buy a full-length pinafore to catch the food that people dropped. I wanted to write a reminder to myself, but that was out of the question. Should I ask Sophie? She had allocated a fixed amount of time and effort to feeding me. Her patience was already being strained through the realisation that she would have to make further sacrifices.

She reappeared with the cloth, which she dropped untidily on my lap. A few areas were left uncovered but I was in no position to complain. I knew that every notch her irritability was raised I would pay for in spilt food, bangs on the mouth or overloaded spoonfuls. It wasn't that she did it intentionally. The next few mouthfuls, each one excessively large, were taken without mishap. Then her friend Jemima arrived.

'Hi, Soph!' She breezed in.

'Hi, Mima,' Soph replied, with a giggle on finding she had withdrawn the spoon too quickly. I felt the tea-towel slide to the floor and I was at risk again from the tablespoon suspended in front of my face. As she conducted her conversation with Jemima she began making patterns in the air with the spoon, like a sparkler on bonfire night.

The strain of coping with her unpredictable attempts to dock the spoon in my mouth and worrying about the renewed exposure of my legs was excruciating. Yet again, I gave way to the conflict between wanting other people to see to my needs and at the same time wishing to be independent. I had been getting fed on and off for a couple of years: why the hell had no one bought me a pinafore? I quickly mellowed and decided to ask for one for my birthday. A pinafore and a straw seemed to be the two most useful aids for this handicap.

With great care and tact, Sophie and I re-established rapport and I was able to enjoy six glorious mouthfuls. We were both laughing, but not for long. It wasn't that I had been brought up to finish everything on my plate, but rather had a need to try to complete projects instead of always having to leave them unfinished. So when Sophie began to take the plate away and I could see that, with judicious scraping, a whole spoonful could still be collected, I began to shake with frustration at not having finished and being unable to say what I wanted.

I blurted out, 'Could you please give. . . ? Finish it!'

' "Could I please fish for it?" '

I was now bouncing in my seat. 'No – finish it.'

'I don't get what you're saying.'

I gave up. 'Yoghurt, please,' I asked.

As she pulled open the fridge I began to smile with the memory of being trapped at the end of a street in Liverpool when I had been caught out watching a gang of teddy boys who were looking as outrageous as possible to attract attention.

'Wharrayuluckina?' one of them shouted, and another grabbed hold of me and said, 'Whatsyername lar?'

'Charles Ivan Vaughan.'

'That's a funny name,' he said. 'Charles Knife and Fork!'

Soph came over with the yoghurt and asked me what I was laughing at. The laughter had unblocked all my tension and I had no difficulty telling her the story. She smiled. I can't say I enjoyed eating the yoghurt, but there was some satisfaction in managing to get it at all. Sophie plonked the spoon in the not quite empty yoghurt pot and dashed off.

'See you Dad.'

'Thanks, Soph.'

I meant it. It wasn't easy to feed me. I often expected a totally unreasonable standard of care. Then I felt a thud on my knee as the heavy tablespoon tipped over the carton and splashed yoghurt over my trousers on its way to the floor.

The Lecture

It was due to start at two o'clock and, because the first dose of the day had the best effect, I had held off taking anything until half an hour before. It was difficult to judge the right moment. If the drug took effect too soon, part of the benefit was wasted. If I left it too late, as the deadline approached I ran the risk of panic drawing me into a whirlpool of fear and failure. My overriding principle was to keep the dose to a minimum. I knew about the side-effects that might develop and my aim was to manage my drug-taking successfully.

I had only half an hour and I was flat on my bed struggling to block out thoughts and images that clamoured for expression. I had to fob them off with assurances that they wouldn't have to wait long, although secretly I knew that they mustn't be allowed to get through at all. I tried breathing deeply and slowly, repeating 'Relax' to myself. The barrier that provided grew in strength and my mind wandered.

I pictured myself in the middle of the night, many years ago, wheeling Sophie backwards and forwards in an old wooden cot. She was on the point of crying. Putting my head near hers, I started short jerky breaths to correspond with her agitated breathing and gradually I drew her into increasingly deeper, more rhythmical breathing. I continued until the new state had carried over into her dreams.

– Oh hell, it's twenty to two and I'm worse than ever.

I struggled to get my hands into a palms-upright position. The effort wrecked my breathing, which came in fast, short gasps. My ankles began to ache with the rigidity that was soaking up the tremor from other limbs. It was a vicious circle. To get calm, I had to stop the tremor; to stop the tremor, I had to get calm. A student had climbed over the wall of my mental barrier and I could see her opening her notebook in readiness. I couldn't help reflect on the different ways she and I would be spending the next fifteen minutes.

Quarter to two and a dialogue began in my head.

– What does it matter if you're a bit late?

– Go away. I don't need you yet.

I knew that once I allowed myself to accept the possibility of being late and to make allowances for pushing the deadline back, I would reduce my commitment to correspond with this extension and stretch out the task to the time available.

– I only came to help you.

– Can't you see I can't put up with any interruptions while there's still hope?

– Yes, but you've got yourself in such a state that if you can see that it's not all that important you may be able to calm down.

– Beat it!

Fluency returned to my ankles; the drugs were beginning to take.

Simultaneously, a variety of images skimmed past my awareness. A bathful of water made sucking noises of protest as it disappeared down the plug hole; a large room full of the noisy, chaotic sounds of partygoers fell silent on the arrival of my famous friend John; the memory of a film in which a vast army of marching ants, finding their way blocked by water, cut leaves off bushes and used them as rafts to get to the other side . . .

– It's through.

I pulled my knees up to my chin, stretched my hands in the air, splayed my fingers apart, stretched my legs straight out and checked that there were sufficient resources to allow independent action of all my limbs.

I leapt off the bed. Seven minutes to go: I'd easily make it. I belted downstairs and through to the back door. A strangely quiet, but very insistent, request pushed forwards into consciousness.

– Oh no!

– I'm sorry, but I've been holding back all morning. I will only take a minute, I promise.

I let go of the door handle, turned round and dashed back upstairs, let my trousers fall to my ankles, sat down and evacuated my bowels in one fell swoop. Quickly use the bidet, up with my trousers, back downstairs and out to the car.

– Hell, you'd better start!

Turn the ignition, pump the accelerator.

– Come on, come on!

– Why did you take the risk and not pump harder?

– I dunno. Anyway, it's going now.

– Don't risk Union Road. Go to the end of Panton Street and use the main road.

Along past the Station Road roundabout, over the bridge. I see the green traffic light and my way is clear down the short stretch of road to college. I know I'm going to make it. The challenge to my reliability has been beaten off until another day. I march confidently down the gravel path, through the glass doors and into the lecture theatre. The racket from a hundred and fifty gossiping first-year students subsides.

'Can I introduce myself?'

Am I sure I don't need notes? It didn't even occur to me to bring any. Interesting that: I usually bring something to fall back on. This was my first lecture to this year group and I felt more confident than ever.

'I've been studying "Motivation and Emotion" for a number of years so I may forget that some concepts are difficult to understand. As I go along, if you don't understand something, just signal and I'll explain in more detail.'

An hour and a half had been timetabled for the lecture, so there was plenty of room for flexibility and even for questions at the end. I was surprised to discover that within ten minutes the lecture had begun to take the form of a discussion.

I asked if anyone could give an example of how their motivation for doing something had been undermined through the intervention of other people. A number of students mentioned the way their parents had offered bribes for keeping up music practice. One student said that her interest in making jewellery as a hobby fell off once she had begun to sell it. Others gave examples where the opposite had happened. I suggested that rewards could increase motivation or undermine it, depending on the circumstances. A student suggested that one's attitude towards the person providing the reward might be an important factor.

'Can you expand on that?' I asked. I waited to give her a chance to formulate a reply. The seconds passed by. I didn't mind; the students seemed to be with me. There was none of the usual coughing and shifting to end the embarrassment of silence. I felt I could hold out even longer. The student suggested that it might depend on whether the recipient of the reward felt that the provider had earned the right to intervene.

Someone asked if all motivation had an emotional component and we developed the idea of a mismatch between aims and achievement which could produce emotional discomfort. The extent to which emotion was involved depended on the extent to which a person had become committed to an activity in terms of caring about its outcome or according to the effort expended. The sense of satisfaction we experience on completing a task might result from an increased flow of energy triggered by a release of chemical transmitters in the brain.

I thought of Freud's account of his experiences on cocaine and the energy that he sensed flowing through his nervous system. I wondered whether cocaine might work to alleviate the symptoms of Parkinson's. I must have taken buckets of L-dopa to get ready for this lecture and now I was beginning to take off, simultaneously processing ideas to select those for inclusion and those to be retained for future reference.

One of the books I'd read on Parkinson's had mentioned how L-dopa had encouraged some patients to embark on highly extravagant, unrealistic projects. My difficulty now was to avoid being seduced by a particularly interesting idea which might irrevocably sidetrack the session with spiralling controversy and complexity.

While keeping a firm grip on the discussion, my mind was busy making links between my illness and the way my ideas about educational theory reflected the cornerstone of my system of values – openness. I sifted through what I was experiencing for ideas with which to check and revise my model of human nature.

I winged up to connect the content of the lecture with the model I was building, but started to see relevance in the very process of connecting between the two levels. At one moment my thoughts served as a context for evaluating the content of the lecture; at the next moment there was a reversal and the content of the lecture served to evaluate the model. But what was I to make of this spiralling of thought to ever more abstract levels? Was the complexity of thinking due to a higher frequency of neural firing in the brain?

I felt it would be a pity if the students were constrained from joining in because they were busy taking notes, so I offered to write a summary and make copies available. It worked well. More students participated in the discussion for the first time. I had a feeling of elation, similar to the effect of anoxia, from the rarefied heights of speculation!

The first hint that it might be time to conclude the session came when I saw a student looking sideways at the clock. We had been going for just over an hour and a half. Simultaneously, I felt the first signs of impending loss of muscular control. Had cues to finish gone unnoticed until collapse was imminent?

I had about ten minutes' grace before the symptoms became severe. I found a good point to bring the lecture to an end and, afraid to risk the walk from the lecture theatre to the main building, I plonked down in a chair and hoped the students would go. A queue formed. I couldn't possibly cope. It would be a pity to ruin the panache of my performance by an exhibition of total collapse. I stood up and told them I was sorry but I was going to have to sit quietly and relax – could they jot down their questions and raise them the following week?

A couple of minutes later I was alone, struggling to impose some control upon the violent shaking by blocking out the temptation to rehearse the lecture to confirm that it really had been a success. For some minutes I battled with worries that another lecture might be due to start at any moment, but finally I was calm, sitting there alone, staring vacantly into space.

The Dewdrop

We piled through the door into the awful neon glare of the Dewdrop. It was probably the best example of bad taste in pub décor in town. This ensured that it was hardly ever crowded. Joyce, behind the bar, was able to feign fierceness but was gentle by nature and would join in our jokes.

Over the past couple of months she'd asked after me. ''Ere, whatever happened to that lovely boy you used to bring in. You know the one who . . .'

I was trembling as my friend Phil told her that they'd brought me to see her in the hope that she might be able to get rid of the awful shaking I had.

'Give him a game of darts. That'll cure him,' she cried. I took her at her word and by rescheduling the tremor to other limbs, managed to serve as a plausible partner in a game of doubles. Then we moved over to a corner of the room and sat there chatting. I decided to take some medication and within half an hour felt it beginning to smooth out the dislocated jerks. Without thinking, I called Joyce to come over.

'We've been wondering, Joyce, if you might have some magic healing powers. About six months ago you accidentally touched Phil and as we were walking home he said that his sore throat had gone. We were wondering if you would have a go on me?'

'I'll do anything you like,' she said.

'I've heard that the best thing is if you face one another with your elbows on the table and press against each other's hands,' said John Ahier.

'Yes, I've heard that,' I said. I was struggling to keep the tremor going by thinking arousing thoughts. We got into position and Joyce had a hard time trying to maintain contact with my dancing fingers.

'It's a sort of magnetism, Joyce. Some people have it, some don't – and we reckon you've got it. Just keep chasing his fingers and when you touch the right one try to keep contact for as long as possible,' said Phil.

'It's like "the Force", Joyce,' said John.

Joyce sat there, clearly concentrating hard on the task she'd been set.

'Wowzer! It's working. I can feel it working!' I cried out.

Soon my hands and fingers were still. Joyce just sat there and eventually said: 'Oh my God!'

'You've done it!' cried Phil. 'Can I bring my sister? She caught this strange incurable disease when she went to Africa.'

'I dunno,' said Joyce. 'I don't understand these things.' She stood up and backed towards the bar. I suggested we have a proper game of darts before the drug wore off.

We noticed her sneaking glances in my direction as she checked up on me, watching the complete fluency and control of my movements and my accuracy at darts. Then we told her what we'd done, and we all collapsed laughing as she bent over the bar thwacking everyone with her folded newspaper – taking care, strangely, not to hit me.

Hypnosis and Other Alternatives

A few years earlier I had read *The Natural History of the Mind* by Gordon Rattray Taylor, which included a brief discussion on hypnosis. It occurred to me that an excellent test of whether my disorder had a functional or a structural basis would be to put me into a deep hypnotic trance and implant a post-hypnotic suggestion that I do something requiring a high degree of muscular control. If after being brought out of the hypnotic state I was able to do it without the usual tremor, this would suggest that the fault was functional rather than structural.

I was excited by the idea and wrote to Taylor to see if he could suggest an expert in hypnosis who might be willing to carry out some serious investigation with me. I wondered if I would be able to achieve the level of control necessary to be taken into a deep hypnotic state, but I pushed this doubt into the background. To my delight, Taylor replied to my letter, suggesting I contact a hypnotist named Lilly Cornfield, who lived in London. I phoned her at once.

I arrived for my first appointment in the huge ground-floor room of a large terraced house in Hampstead. After a brief chat Lilly, who looked like a female version of Bertrand Russell, asked me to lie on a bed and close my eyes. She began to mutter indistinctly, then passed her hands over my chest and arms, held my head and carried out a variety of other manoeuvres.

At the end of the session I managed with some difficulty to ask if that had been hypnosis. She said she would do hypnosis next time if I liked, so I made another appointment. I wasn't at all clear what she had been trying to do during this first session. I raised the question of payment and she generously left it to me. I gave her a modest sum, thanked her very much and left. I was deeply disappointed, suspecting that whatever happened next time would still be a far cry from those discreet changes in state that I had seen on television. I kept up my visits, however, in the ever-diminishing hope that this apprenticeship would be followed by the real thing. Lighted candles appeared round the bed and I began to feel that Lilly's aim was to exorcise demons from my body. Sadly, I concluded that I was not going to be able to test my hypothesis and my visits dropped off.

I contacted a Cambridge physiotherapist named Harry 'Killer' Willis to check if the cause of the illness might have been either a pulled muscle or a slipped disc. I wondered if the chemical resources for keeping muscles under control had been syphoned off to cope while the damage repaired itself. If the damage could be put right by some form of manipulation or physiotherapy, these scarce resources might become available again for sharing out. The loss of control in my muscles would then disappear.

Harry had had years of experience manipulating the backs and muscles of sportsmen and athletes who had injured themselves. I cycled over to his house, hoping he would give me a thorough examination and would find a serious abnormality around the base of the spine. When I had mentioned these ideas to Iain Wilkinson he had listened courteously but had not made any suggestion for further action.

'Oh, you've got Parkinson's disease,' said Harry as soon as he saw me. 'There's no need to check your back.'

He told me about his training, which had included throwing medicine balls at patients with Parkinson's disease. I also knew that he had taken up hypnosis as a hobby, so I mentioned my interest in it and he offered to do some sessions with me free of charge.

He allocated me a slot in his weekly appointments and we met regularly. I would lie down and Harry would gently guide me from high to low levels of arousal. He would describe scenes of calm: for example, he might suggest that I was lying on a grassy slope high in an Alpine pasture, enjoying the warmth from the sun and watching the gentle gliding of birds in the valley below. Harry was very generous and kind and I enjoyed the times we spent together, but what about the deep trance? If this was hypnosis, it seemed very weak and watery. Eventually I stopped the sessions, as I felt that they weren't moving beyond the preliminary stages.

A Cambridge party can be an extraordinary affair. If you have an illness, it is very likely there will be someone there who knows a wizard or genius for dealing with your particular complaint. It was at a party that I was given the name of a qualified doctor who was very interested in hypnosis. She was Dr Rosemary Summers, who had fairly recently completed her medical training. I rang her and suggested that she might find me an interesting case.

Rosemary came round to my house and we discussed the best way to proceed. It wasn't difficult for her to convince me that there should be no fee involved since it was going to be an experiment for herself as much as for me. It wasn't that I was mean about paying for time and expertise, but I didn't want to go back on my principle of not wanting to obtain medical help of a special kind simply because I could pay for it. I also felt a need to avoid appearing foolish by having wasted a lot of money if nothing came of these excursions into alternative medicine.

Rosemary's approach was similar to Harry's, though she was more systematic. She was also eager to try out a couple of tapes of hypnotic exercises she had had sent from America. They induced a state of calm through visual and auditory settings of peacefulness, and on a couple of occasions I fell asleep. I realised how the states of sleep and relaxation differed; there was no guarantee that during sleep the mental apparatus would be relaxed.

I still wasn't reaching the deep-trance state that I sought; nevertheless, I began to think that there was something in the technique of relaxing which might be beneficial. Although I wasn't able to demonstrate a return to complete muscular control after I'd come out of the hypnotic state, I was managing to remove all signs of tremor during the course of relaxation. Rosemary and I agreed that what we were doing was similar to meditation. I remembered a postcard that Paul McCartney had sent from India with its picture of the Maharishi Yogi. Then it had required some effort to keep an open mind that beneath the mumbo-jumbo and personality cult there might be something worthwhile.

Rosemary was friendly with someone involved with an organisation for promoting meditation in this country. She arranged for us both to visit the centre. When the day came, I took my drugs soon after setting out and as usual went into a worse state immediately prior to the process of synthesis and allocation in the brain. As we approached the long drive through the estate to the main building I asked Rosemary to stop so that I could swing up and down on the bars of the gate to try to induce the drugs to work. I wondered if it was the excitement that was somehow affecting them; perhaps they hadn't been processed in the gut and the chemical wasn't even in the bloodstream yet? Or perhaps it was in the bloodstream and my state was inhibiting its passage across the blood–brain barrier? Maybe it was in the brain and had been synthesised to dopamine but was being syphoned from muscular control to other functions? Was the L-dopa being converted to dopamine outside the brain? The increase in excitability could then be explained by the stimulating action that I assumed dopamine to have upon the heart.

I was still shaking when I got back into the car and we drove up to the front of the huge old Victorian mansion. I hobbled in behind Rosemary, upset that I might not get a chance to impress the people who were our hosts and whom I hoped to persuade to do some research on the relationship between meditation and Parkinson's.

They showed us round. I was fascinated by the 'flying room' – a large area covered with a massive blue mattress. They showed us photographs of people a foot or so in the air. I wasn't sure what to think. They admitted it wasn't really flying but rather a sporadic bouncing which was achieved only after a great deal of practice!

They had a couple of people conducting research into meditation. I was excited to get my ideas across, and maybe this arousal finally induced the drugs to take, but I got the impression that they were being patient while I spoke rather than interested in what I said. I felt rather disappointed as we drove away. They had suggested that I undertake a course of meditation to see if it improved my symptoms. I thought that the technique might be useful but, like the spa towns with their expensive hotels and exploitation of simple spring water, meditation had been packaged and mystified and used to amass wealth and property. Perhaps, though, I could gain some benefit from relaxation techniques without being exploited.

My problem was that my actions were subject to interference from shaking, so what I needed was something to interfere with the interference and stop the tremor. It had to be something that would not excite me, something that would work at a moment's notice and cut through whatever my current experience happened to be. One obvious possibility was the use of a mantra. I found that a single word was inadequate since it was too easy to repeat it while simultaneously carrying on with my other thoughts and preoccupations.

It was out of the question to try to stop the brain thinking – all one could hope to do was to preoccupy it with emotion-free nonsense. The brain would use every trick imaginable to throw off this imposition and therefore it was essential to find a phrase which was not so difficult that the mind became interested in it. I came across a religious mantra in *The Snow Leopard*: 'Om mani padme hum'. I decided that I wanted to get away from religious connotations and I hit upon the title of one of Mozart's operas, *Idomeneo*. Then I added the word 'hum' to achieve the balance and rhythm of the original Tibetan mantra. When I tried it, however, I found it was too simple: I was able to think about other things at the same time as repeating it. So I made it more complicated by inserting numbers; this led to the final version, 'Idomen one two eo hum three four five Idomen six seven eo hum eight nine ten Idomen . . .'. That is just about the right level to occupy my mind, blocking out anxious thoughts yet not so difficult in itself that it uses up resources.

In time this chant became extremely useful in stopping panic in its tracks, in triggering a boost to the flow of resource when I was stuck in bed at night, and in numerous other situations. To my surprise, it also worked for recalling people's names.

Hypnosis had not been a waste of time after all. There was also tangible benefit for Rosemary in the form of a paper delivered to a society for medical hypnosis at a meeting held at the Royal Society in London. I enjoyed taking part and answering questions concerning the limits and the possibilities of hypnosis for Parkinson's.

The urgency to find an alternative to L-dopa became greater when I began to experience some of its adverse reactions. The tremor was certainly quelled by the drugs, but after a few months muscle twitching broke out in my face. My moods swung unaccountably from happy conviviality to intolerant irritation. I was horrified on one occasion to have lost my temper and hit Sophie. Was there a way I could get the chemical inside me through a slow rate of absorption rather than in sudden bursts?

In the library I had come across a couple of papers which mentioned that the seeds of a plant, *Mucuna puriens*, which grew in South America where its seeds were used by the native Indians as aphrodisiacs, contained L-dopa. I visited the library at the Botanic Garden nearby and obtained the addresses of gardens which had these seeds on their lists for swapping. I also discovered that L-dopa occurred naturally in fava beans, which were used by the bucket load as pig-feed in the United States. My request for Mucuna seeds was unsuccessful but I discovered that Arjuna, a local health-food shop, had plenty of fava beans. I had beans on their own, beans in stews – enough beans, I felt sure, to provide the same amount of L-dopa as I took in the tablets. I was full of beans but still not jumping! The lack of any noticeable effect left us with the problem of how to use up the huge sack of beans in the cupboard.

While I was still trying out the beans, Margaret Schofield, the beautifully supple Cambridge yoga teacher, offered to conduct a few sessions with me; she too waived any fee. She had me twisting and bending and, most important of all, breathing correctly. She remarked on the shallowness with which I breathed, but in spite of her instructions I found it extraordinarily difficult to fill my lungs and stomach with air. There was nothing in the literature which said breathing was implicated in the Parkinson deficit, yet I noticed a regular mechanical interplay between the tremor in my limbs and breathing. The more deeply I breathed, the greater the tremor. Were the muscles for the lungs served by the same system as the muscles in the arms and legs?

During the sessions with Margaret I managed to increase the fluency of my movements but was left in the same, or possibly a worse, state afterwards. It was as if the induction, through setting up demand, could not be matched by the supply of resources.

I also tried Shiatsu with a woman called Rhea. This entailed locating and stimulating particular pressure points, followed by relaxation. I think these pressure points were supposed to be linked in some hierarchical fashion to form a channel for energy to flood through the system. The feet seemed to be an important junction from which the flow of energy radiated out to other parts. I was impressed by Rhea's serenity, even when she stood on me with her feet balanced on either side of my body!

It was very difficult to be sure whether an apparent interaction between my symptoms, the drugs and the food I ate was due to anything other than chance. I got the impression that eating fish for supper affected how good I felt in the early morning, when I tried to manage on storage of the chemical from the previous day. Tea seemed to make me very restless in bed at night. On a couple of occasions, the time when I'd taken the drug and felt highly nauseated seemed to be very close to drinking coffee. Raisins at breakfast seemed to delay the drugs taking. Alcohol seemed to have an effect, but I could never be sure whether this was beneficial or detrimental at different phases of its absorption. Champagne seemed to enhance storage! I contacted the Dunn Nutritional Research Unit in Cambridge, but could find nobody who was interested in investigating scientifically possible links between diet and Parkinson's.

In spite of the seemingly unpredictable nature of the symptoms, I remained convinced that they were not arbitrary and I felt sure that I could still make some headway in revealing the laws that governed them.

My Sister Bernice

'Bernice insane – at risk – action essential.'

Shaking violently, I dropped the telegram on to the table. My sister's neighbours had decided to step up the pressure by using shock tactics. They were likely to succeed. I got calm again by trying to see their point of view. For months now there had been phone calls and correspondence about Bernice's deteriorating behaviour.

She'd had schizophrenia for eighteen years, but the family's policy of encouraging her to live independently had succeeded up till now. We had been helped in this by the generosity of one of my friends, who put up the money for a flat in London close to where I used to live. For a while Bernice had a job in a library. She managed on her own and was very reluctant to take the medication prescribed for her illness. There were all sorts of adverse effects from the drugs; for example, a compulsion to smoke an enormous number of cigarettes and a Parkinson-type tremor which I'd been very distressed to see long before the genuine Parkinson's broke out in me.

There had been a number of crises over the years but these had not lasted long and had been tolerated by her neighbours. This time, however, her shouting and her insistence on having her radio and television playing loudly day and night had gone too far. The noisy tramp up and down the stairs of the teenagers she invited to tea had finally goaded the neighbours to get together to have Bernice moved out for good. We did understand what they had to put up with and I was becoming ever more convinced that she would have to leave.

It was a hopeless situation. Bern refused to go to see the doctor and get medication. There were injections that would last over a couple of months if only she could be persuaded, tricked or bribed into having them, but then there were the side-effects. A complex moral dilemma hung around the business of her medication. She was happy enough without drugs; there were no indications of suffering of any kind that we could use to delude ourselves into thinking the medication was for the sake of her happiness. The drugs made her feel sick. They also brought her back to a reality that she was unable to face. But without them her behaviour was a severe disturbance to her neighbours. The only conclusion that it was possible to reach was that Bern must take the medication as a means of social control.

I responded to the telegram by promising to do what I could. I arranged a meeting between the social services, the neighbours, their solicitor and myself, but my confidence was shattered when I discovered that because the flats were leasehold, the freeholders (one of the major building societies) could demand forfeiture of the lease and liquidated damages.

The correspondence and meetings had dragged on for four years. Now I finally caved in and took action through the County Court to secure Bern's eviction. She was adamant about not moving and this was the only way we could avoid forfeiting the lease and a considerable loss of money.

It was a miserable, wet day as the social worker, my other sister Anne, Bern and I filed into Court Number 1 at Clerkenwell. I hadn't a clue about procedures, but to save money had chosen to conduct my own case. The magistrate's clerk decided he couldn't deal with the case and arranged for it to be considered by a judge later in the day.

It soon became apparent what a complete shambles the proceedings were going to be. I went up to the witness box to present my case and was immediately asked by the judge: 'Where are your witnesses?'

'I don't have any.'

'But you've got to have witnesses,' he exploded. At that moment the neighbour who had sent the telegram entered the court to observe the outcome and in a flash I called her to be my witness.

'Are you willing to be a witness?' cried the judge. She nervously replied that she hadn't intended it but was willing if it would help.

As it became clear that the case was going to begin, Bern stood up and started shouting across the court in her own defence.

'Your Honour, Your Almighty, or whatever you call yourself, there is no case to answer. I'm a perfectly law-abiding policewoman, trained by the BBC, and instructed specifically to live in that flat to ensure that the war that's going on all around us doesn't get out of hand. There is absolutely no case to answer, Your Worship. I can tell you categorically now that there are no grounds for my leaving the flat. I rule this case out of order! In the name of the Law and the Virgin Birth, no one has any right to move me out of that flat. We're all dupes and there have been hundreds of times in past lives when I've lived in that flat. Your Honour, we have to keep the concept alive . . .'

Throughout Bern's shouting the judge threatened to have her

removed and called on her to sit down. Bill, a social worker who had generously added Bernice to his case-load, struggled to quieten her and keep her under control. I was beginning to fall apart all over the witness stand, shaking and trembling, and I could see the judge going through an agonising reappraisal of the situation. His extreme irritation gave way to understanding and he began to bend the rules in order to get the case dealt with. He prompted me with the questions I should ask my witness.

'Yes, and now don't you want to ask about the noise and whether there was any banging of windows?'

'Oh yes,' I said and turned to the witness. 'And was there banging of windows and a lot of noise?'

'And did this go on throughout the night?' added the judge, inviting me to extend my question.

'There is absolutely no case to answer,' Bern shouted.

'Sit down.'

'You're not a real judge, you're just a dupe. There's a war on, isn't there?'

The hearing muddled its way along, eating a great chunk out of the judge's lunchtime, but he seemed determined to get shot of the case and not have it drag on all afternoon.

I obtained the eviction order to be implemented a month later. The eviction so disturbed Bern that it led to police involvement in her admission to the psychiatric wing of the nearby hospital, where she had to stay until she agreed to take the drugs. For the past two years she has been living in a short-stay hostel run by the social services. Two or three times a year she ends up in hospital for a course of treatment.

One might conclude that the best solution would be to find some means of convincing her to take her medication voluntarily – but all our attempts failed. While she was still living in the flat I remember spending three or four hours at the doctor's getting her to the point of having an injection which she rejected at the last minute. As I drove her home she started shouting in response to the voices that filled her consciousness. To my shame, I gave in to my frustration and smacked her on the arm. I stopped the car and made her walk the rest of the way home.

I was being totally unfair. Her doctors had just raised her drugs to what they called a 'therapeutic' level, arguing that the previous dosage was ineffective. This increase worried me a great deal. No one understood better than I her right to refuse the drugs, and yet I was furious that she wouldn't accept them.

Although there is no evidence that Parkinson's disease and schizophrenia are linked, one can't help but speculate on the contrasts between the two illnesses. Whereas my disease has produced a loss of muscular control, her illness results in a profound disturbance of thought and emotion. She suffers from a breakdown in the mental processes by which we differentiate our inner self from the outside world. Her innermost thoughts, feelings and acts seem to be known to, or caused by, other people, organisations, natural or unnatural forces. Professor Marsden suggests that Parkinson patients suffer a breakdown in the execution of learned plans.

Bernice's mind seems possessed by involuntary forces in a similar way to my body. The interesting thing is that whereas my brain lacks dopamine, people diagnosed as schizophrenic suffer an excess of dopamine. The difference is that whereas Parkinson's disease is due to a destruction of part of the brain, there is, as yet, no identifiable damage or disease process which causes the excess dopamine in Bernice's brain.

The awful irony is that the drugs Bernice has been given have produced Parkinsonian symptoms. Adverse reactions to the drugs are now permanent and irreversible. The early tremor has been replaced by dyskinesia. Her hands writhe continually and control over her facial muscles has collapsed.

I don't know what else I could have done in the circumstances. I believe in my right to manage my own drugs, and yet I acted against Bernice because she wouldn't take hers.

Letter to Professor Marsden

I reached a stage, four years after discovering I had Parkinson's, where I was disillusioned with my research in schools. Faced with the prospect of analysing the data and writing up, I decided to abandon my Ph.D. and to concentrate instead on summarising my findings on Parkinson's. I wanted to send a copy of my summary to Professor Marsden.

My first aim was simply to purge my mind of the frequent repetition and rediscovery of connections between different aspects of Parkinson's, and of the effects of L-dopa on aspects of my life and personality. I was excited about these ideas, but at the same time felt hesitant about sending such disjointed speculations to someone as eminent as Professor Marsden.

Nevertheless, I was used to this role of David taking on Goliath and no harm could be done, except to my ego if he ignored me. I took encouragement from the fact that Professor Marsden had replied to a previous letter asking him to recommend a book that would explain the current level of knowledge about Parkinson's in language I would be able to understand. He had recommended an excellent book by an American, Professor Duvoisin, entitled *Parkinson's Disease. A guide for patient and family*. I went through it with a fine-tooth comb, checking to see if my experience contradicted anything it said. I decided to send a copy of my summary to Duvoisin as well, hoping that he might recognise the value of the point I was making and would then feel like commenting on the rest.

A third copy went to Professor Karl Pribram at Stanford University, whom I admired for the way in which he successfully combined expertise in neuro-physiology with a deep understanding of psychology and attempted to bridge the gulf between the two, even publishing his speculations before much scientific evidence had been collected.

After about ten days I still had not heard from any of them, so I went through what I had written. It seemed reasonable enough and there were a number of ideas which I was sure were original. I pushed it into the background and occupied myself with other things, persuading myself that it was not that important, although in fact it was the culmination of months of careful observation and monitoring.

The truth was that I had invested an enormous amount of myself in the supportive research behind what I had written. I had had to sort through notes scattered on bits of paper, notebooks and anything that had happened to be handy at the time. I had written it while off the drugs, relying on a good level of storage, since this was the state in which I could summon the greatest degree of clarity for analysis. I thought it was one of my more valuable discoveries that the level of take-up of L-dopa by the body not only affected muscular control but also the quality of thought, particularly the difference between analysis and creativity.

I was so convinced of the importance of what I had written that I expected the three professors to drop all their commitments in order to reply immediately! One week would be a reasonable time to wait for a reply, I thought; two weeks would suggest it was of secondary importance; and any longer would mean it didn't deserve a reply at all.

Three weeks had passed when Jan came into my bedroom one morning with a letter, saying: 'This has come for you.' I looked at the postmark and wondered who would be writing to me from London. Who did I know from SE5? I handed it back to Jan because my hands had started to shake as my curiosity was aroused. I still had no idea whom the letter was from. Jan opened it and handed it to me; we had agreed not to let my illness take away the pleasure of being the first to read my own post. I read the words 'Maudsley Hospital' – it was from Professor Marsden.

I had tried to stop thinking about the possibility of a reply and had been wondering what other projects I might take on. In his first sentence, however, Professor Marsden talked about my letter greeting him from a trip abroad and I forgot at once all the excuses and explanations I'd mustered to explain the delay. The excitement I felt quickly made obvious all the emotion and tension I had been suppressing, the amount of time and effort I had spent and the importance to me of his opinion of my discoveries.

'Oh Jan, listen to this – he finds my ideas about the cause of the illness interesting! He wants to hear about the way food and drink affect how the drug works.' I skimmed over the paragraphs looking for key phrases – and there they were: ' "I am most interested in your observations on the effect of sleep. . . . I am intrigued . . . I am also very interested . . ." ' – Jan, listen, he says he's intrigued by my notion of different sorts of sleep influencing transmitter availability. He thinks it's worth doing research on it. He says he'd like to hear my views on the way in which, when I'm stuck unable to move at all, perception and emotion might change. Jan, he wants me to go down and talk with him!'

Jan said she was pleased for me. She had put up with a lot, particularly when I went off the drugs for periods of up to a week. I hoped she agreed that it had all been worthwhile; I wasn't sure, but she repeated how glad she was that I'd received such a super letter. She knew from experience that if I felt I could get away with it, I would come off the drugs for a month. She had had to tolerate me falling all over the place and going totally rigid before. So I knew she would be careful about dropping her guard and being too enthusiastic about my experiments.

I didn't even consider whether I should delay making an appointment in case my eagerness put Professor Marsden off. I rang through to his secretary and arranged to see him at ten o'clock the following Wednesday.

That day I caught the eight o'clock train from Cambridge to Liverpool Street Station. The drugs had taken in good time and I was able to use the resultant fluency to read through the ten pages of closely typed notes I'd sent to Professor Marsden.

It was as if I'd sent a chapter of a thesis to my supervisor and now had to be sure that I could back up what I'd said and not just fizzle out at the viva! I'd made the bold statement that memory retrieval is improved with L-dopa. It was in fact much more complicated than that, and I was a bit worried that by the time the meeting took place I might have moved into a further phase of the effects of L-dopa where I became reduced to a rather bland state. It was going to be difficult to time things right.

I read through the section I had written on causes, which was where I had described my pet theory. The key point was that various sources of stress might compound to produce a catastrophic breakdown under particular circumstances. My hypothesis centred on cells becoming exhausted by over-production of dopamine to meet unusually high levels of compound stress. In that state of low resistance, poisoning of the dopamine-producing cells in the brain might occur.

In his letter Professor Marsden had picked up on the idea that particular stressful activities – alcohol, exercise and intercourse – made impossible demands on dopaminergic cells. So if you already had Parkinson's, alcohol and exercise (including intercourse) could make the symptoms worse. What he didn't pick up was my idea that these activities could, in certain circumstances, combine to trigger the onset of the disease.

I now started searching my letter for other things he hadn't mentioned.

I must remember to tell him about putting my back out and what a fright it gave me. Then I can describe the mad way I did weightlifting to make sure my back didn't give way again.

One of the early symptoms of Parkinson's can be numbness in the limbs. He says alcohol affects the symptoms but he doesn't comment on the fact that for years I used to get feelings of numbness when I drank. He'll say millions of people drink and don't get Parkinson's, but my argument is not that alcohol in itself causes the disease, but in combination with other factors, it may contribute to creating a state which predisposes Parkinson's. Remember that guy who had been drinking spirits all evening, went for a walk at three o'clock in the morning on a freezing cold night and had a stroke. The body can only compensate for so much before collapsing under the strain.

I must avoid giving him the impression that I'm preoccupied with sex, but it's puzzling the way it's played down in Duvoisin's book.

I must try to get over the remarkable threefold coincidence of the same factors cropping up influencing the symptoms, being influenced by the drugs and presenting themselves among possible causes.

I must get clear the way I use the word stress. He'd be right to argue that it is used very loosely. I think what I'll do is distinguish between the different kinds of source which may initiate stress – muscular for weightlifting, socio-psychological for adhering to rules that are difficult to follow, physiological in the case of exposure to cold. The idea is that all these home in on the same area in the brain.

The measure of the severity of the symptoms might be worth raising. I'll have to be careful not to give the impression that I'm trying to question the way they measure severity, simply because I don't want to be pigeon-holed as being in the early, middle or late stage of the disease. If everyone with Parkinson's is supposed to have lost 80 per cent of a particular cluster of brain cells, it seems we are all in a pretty severe state. The best way to distinguish between individuals might be to see how quickly and with what amounts of L-dopa they could be brought back to full control. Another possibility might be to see how long it takes after stopping the drugs for a person to lose the benefit of his storage and what degree of deficit he shows when he stops deteriorating further.

That's a good point. In my letter I had said:

A person may be able to override resting tremor but the more he does this, the more other thresholds are breached. As these are unkeyed there comes a point where so many functions are being held that moving a limb can no longer be kept smooth by allocating the strain elsewhere.

He says acupuncture has been tried; a pity that. I might press him further on the question of Carbidopa being linked to my toe-nails dying, since I'm sure it affects blood flow.

A pity he doesn't mention relaxation – sorry, he does. Here it is: 'One of the major problems in Parkinson's disease is the fatigue it produces so anything that causes relaxation may allow you to build up a store of transmitter for subsequent use.' I'll try to get him to say how relaxation works, because when off the drug I can still achieve a calm state.

That's a puzzle – my voice going very quiet after the L-dopa has taken. A pity he's ignored circadian rhythms and an even greater pity I haven't been able to find much in the literature about them. It does seem that about four or five in the morning is an important time for the release of chemical transmitters in preparation for the tasks of the day ahead.

It's marvellous that he's grasped hold of the topic of sleep. It's taken me months to try to sort that one out. It's probably expecting too much for him to get interested in my speculations about dreaming. It's a lovely discovery that the quality of the dream changes from being unfavourable to favourable in exact correspondence to the chemical coming on stream and flooding the system. One of the best examples of this was being locked into a dream where I was being insulted and injured. About four o'clock I woke up briefly, lay quiet for a while, felt mobility return to my limbs, fell asleep again and resumed the dream where I'd left off. The theme was the same but the tone had changed. It was as if I'd swallowed my tin of spinach and could now take on allcomers – and the dream concluded highly favourably.

I'd love to get a chance to discuss my idea of the links between dreaming and depression:

Dreaming in the early morning depletes the amount of transmitter available for the day's activities. Dreaming affords an opportunity for unfavourable events to be given a favourable emotion. Depression arises when the provision of transmitters is insufficient for blocking off an experience in the first place, or providing a satisfactory conclusion. The attempt to sort out problems through dreams depletes transmitters for the daytime, leading to lethargy. The perception of such lack of energy can exacerbate the situation and lead to greater depression. This would compound the experience of low processing capabilities in respect of thinking.

I hope I get a chance to discuss these ideas about dyskinetic movement. The literature seems to suggest an explanation in terms of hypersensitive receptors being bombarded by excessive dopamine. My impression is that cells serving functions not yet caught up in the deficit lose their normal role as a result of being recruited into the manufacture of dopamine for functions whose cells have broken down. The dyskinesias reflect their temporary exhaustion. This suggests a 'hard-wiring' model for links between cells and functions, and I may be expected to try to reconcile that with my support for the opposite notion of a general pool of dopamine.

I went through Duvoisin's book very carefully to see if there was anything that differed from my own experience; it was exciting to find in his discussion of nausea that the vomiting centre 'regards L-dopa, an unusual substance to find in the circulation, as an offensive material to be thrown out'. I'm sure I'm right on this one. The whole point of Carbidopa is to inhibit the enzyme that destroys L-dopa and allow it to survive in greater quantities. This should reduce sickness because if the enzyme is allowed to do its conversion job, the nausea centre gets triggered by the resulting dopamine flooding the system outside the brain.

I wonder what he'll make of all this speculation where I've outlined a model for dopamine? The stuff seems to play a part in all sorts of things: concentration, dreaming, thinking, creativity, rewarding experience, depression, religious experience – the list is huge.

I wonder how much time we'll have – we'll never get through all this . . .

At the Maudsley Hospital

After a while the heat in the crowded compartment began to have an effect. As we approached London my thoughts quickly abandoned my notes and were concentrated on how to maintain control. It was essential to clear the decks while I could and avoid being left with anything to carry should control be lost. In spite of the heat I stood up and put on my light jacket, folded my notes and stuffed them deep into a pocket. I couldn't risk getting stuck in London during the rush hour so I took some more drugs, hoping I was not too late to overlap with the previous dose. I had allowed myself an hour for getting across London, but as I wandered round the maze of the Elephant and Castle I became more and more anxious that I was going to be late.

'Flippin' deadlines again!' Everything was becoming a deadline. Even in conversation there was a deadline to say what I wanted before the other person assumed I had nothing to contribute and carried on.

Eventually I found the right bus-stop. The appointment was in quarter of an hour and I decided not to take any more drugs so soon after the last dose; I wanted to impress Professor Marsden with the way I was managing the medication, so I didn't want to be overcome by writhing dyskinesias.

At five to ten, still on the bus, I lost control. The conductor shouted out the name of the hospital and I stumbled on to the pavement with hands clasped behind my back to prevent myself falling over. I followed the directions to Professor Marsden's office. I was on time, but my concern to be in a good state and the resulting anxiety had left me shaking violently.

Professor Marsden welcomed me and directed me to a chair. His phone rang immediately. While he answered it I looked round his office and was surprised how modest in size it was for a man with such an important position.

The phone conversation went on for some time. I was desperately keen to regain control, so thought I would illustrate one way I had developed for speeding up the process. I moved from the chair and stretched out on the floor, hands by my sides, palms turned upwards, feet splayed out, eyes closed. I started repeating nonsense to myself and tried to fight back images of how the scene must appear to an outsider – as if Professor Marsden were reporting the discovery of a dead body in his study. Could I muster control before he finished on the phone?

'Idomen one two, eo hum three four five . . .'

It was coming! It was there! I turned my back on Professor Marsden and stretched my arms and fingers to induce the flow of energy into my hands and arms. His phone call finished; he seemed to ignore the various displays I'd carried out. Had he seen it all before?

He sat down and asked me to describe what happened to me when I came off the drug. I launched into a speculative account of what was going on. After a while he interrupted me and said, 'It's facts that we want. Try to give me the facts.'

That's all very well, I said to myself, but the very choice of words for describing the 'facts' creates a bias. I asked if it was all right to use the word 'control' and to describe the problem as to do with losing control.

'Yes, that's all right.'

I persuaded myself that I could understand his emphasis on a factual account and proceeded to tell him about memory and the difficulties of retrieval when off L-dopa giving way to fluent recall after the drugs had worked.

I was disappointed with my performance. As so frequently happened after I had taken my second or third dose, the drugs provided the facility for uttering what I was thinking but there was a damping effect on my ability to sort out the ideas.

Although there may be other factors, the main one in determining whether I'm able to think fluently and creatively is the number of doses I've had so far in any one day. At that time I was also having to accept that the situation was deteriorating. In the early days of taking L-dopa, adverse effects arose far less frequently. For example, if we gave a dinner party it was difficult to choose between staying off the drugs, having to be fed and enjoying myself by succeeding in contributing to the conversation through conserving energy and blurting out witty remarks at key moments, or taking the drugs, only to feel disinclined from joining in at all. The drugs seemed to produce a kind of depression. Maybe they induced a feeling of detachment.

I was very disappointed, and apologised to Professor Marsden for not managing to be clearer in my account. He generously reassured me that, on the contrary, I had described the effects of the illness upon memory very well indeed. I thought for a moment about what it must be like to be in his position. He must be aware that anything he said would carry very considerable authority; consequently he had to be extremely careful. I had always been amused by the careful phraseology used in research papers: 'There is no evidence to support. . . . There is conflicting evidence. . . .' So many false hopes must be raised by premature conclusions based on inconclusive research, although there is, of course, a risk that excessive caution might mean that important research findings are ignored. Professor Marsden refused to speculate – or, more likely, refused to make public the speculations he had.

Shortly after eleven the meeting was over. I offered to take part in any research that he might think worthwhile. Initially, I would be willing to be the subject of experiments devised by him or his research team. Having once secured a foothold I hoped to be able to convince him of the validity of my own proposals. Was I being naïve in thinking that I could succeed in breaking the doctor–patient relationship to become accepted into the medical community on the basis of having knowledge of Parkinson's, which, although non-scientific, might nevertheless be equally valid? I must be careful not to frighten them off through appearing to be too pushy about wanting them to investigate my own hypotheses.

I went back to the Maudsley Hospital on three occasions to do tests to explore more efficient ways of administering L-dopa. On one of the visits I tried to persuade a couple of Professor Marsden's assistants to visit me in Cambridge for a weekend so that I could demonstrate things which I found difficult to illustrate at the hospital. I wanted to be the subject of an individual case-study, the manipulations of the symptoms, drug-taking and interpretative models of which would illuminate many aspects of Parkinson's disease.

Part of me was able to appreciate how dedicated and short of time these people were, but nonetheless I felt it was a pity that nobody came. Nor was there much hope of getting Professor Marsden to turn over part of his research budget and department to investigating my brilliant hypotheses!

Early Morning

– That's odd: it's still pitch dark. How come the birds are singing?

I nudged my arm over the side of the bed and let it drop down to the floor. It remained free of tremor. My fingers picked their way across the carpet to where the clock should have been. My arm was fully stretched but I'd missed the clock.

– Why isn't it there?

I tried not to get stuck in the usual bog of speculation and recrimination. Trembling with the arousal that followed any irritation or frustration, my fingers began to retrace their steps. Curling backwards in readiness, they lunged forwards in a slightly different direction.

I allowed myself a moment's satisfaction that I was succeeding quite well and chopped back interpretations as they sprouted from my subconscious. I knew what was happening; it had all been done with such cunning. By managing to reach for the clock I'd blocked the pathways of interruption and tremor. It was like a duel between the forces of darkness and light. The Devil slowly turned over his trump card and whispered: 'No harm in relishing your success for a minute.' But I was on my guard and resisted the indulgence by playing my ace, 'Idomeneo hum', my mantric warrior. Very soon my mind hummed in soothing peace and my fingers found themselves released from the lock that had held them rigid, stiffly gripping the carpet. Fluency returned to my wrist, elbow and shoulder as the rhythmic nonsense became more and more richly established.

I didn't consciously decide on a new tactic, but had anybody been watching they would have seen my whole arm raised in the air with my body poised along the edge of the bed. Instead of fingers creeping across the carpet, I launched into a large swooping movement in which the clock was caught and carried up to be held in front of my short-sighted eyes.

– Four o'clock. Great! It's nearly daybreak. Those birds are a puzzle though. Perhaps they're jet-lagged from their migration.

For a long time I had noticed an extraordinary boost in muscular fluency which flooded my body sometime around dawn. I'd puzzled over the possible role played by the sun in determining the particular time when this occurred. Could there be a brain mechanism so sensitive to light intensity that it registered changes even through the thick blind over my window? Or could the boost be triggered by a change in temperature? Maybe the roof of the mouth housed some sort of thermometer for measuring the change in temperature of the air breathed in?

I began to get excited by the originality of these ideas. For the time being it didn't matter that they might be absurd. I was pleased to find that I was able to indulge in speculation without any noticeable disturbance to muscular control. It was like surfing on a wave of fluency.

But I'd held the clock too long – the Devil was going to win after all. He'd caught me out. He knew how I loved ruminating on the ways of human nature. Exploiting this, he had pushed me from detached reflection into the emotional excitement of creativity and whispered to his accomplices: 'If he will insist on tackling such an ambitious project as going for that clock we'll entice him by offering him whatever he enjoys most. Then hit him with all the tremor we can muster, and if he holds out against that, we'll freeze him to stone!'

I let my arm drop and just managed to open my fingers before the power of the tremor made it impossible to release my grip. By linking the smooth flow of my dropping arm to letting go of the clock I had managed to harness gravity again to achieve the action I wanted.

I was now wide awake. I tried to judge whether removing the bedclothes would produce a blast of cold air and destroy my ability to get out of bed. The weather forecast had predicted a clear start to the day with frost in places.

– It's likely to be cold. I'm going to have to be quick.

I wasn't going to succeed if I spent too long working out a careful plan: dropping to the floor, placing one hand on the bed, the other on the chair, drawing my left leg forwards and so on. The enormity of the task would weigh too heavily and tremor would break out if I rehearsed the act in my mind's eye. There was another danger of pre-rehearsal – an unexpected event could leave me marooned and unable to reschedule resources from other functions.

Thus, I was on the floor.

– Quick, on your knees!

I grabbed the back of the chair and gripped the bedclothes with my other hand.

– Blast, they're coming loose. Let go!

In one movement I jack-knifed up and reached for the branch of the tree painted on the wall.

– I've done it!

Before my trembling legs had a chance to undo the achievement, I swung my arms behind my back and, with hands clasped to ensure I didn't fall, moved over to the wash-basin. Edging up my track suit after peeing and briefly running the tap, I glanced towards the door in the dim light that now filtered into the room. It looked closed.

– Did I close it? No, it must have been . . . hell, stop it!

I managed to shelve that line of thought and began my soothing ritual movements. Fingers lifted to my shoulder then down to the door handle, back to my shoulder, then to the radiator. Shoulder, radiator, shoulder, radiator, and then a slow-motion pounce for the door handle. Faced with a stream of cool air as the door opened, I started to go rigid.

– Will I be able to tackle Grantchester this morning? The 'four-mile marathon'!

I noted my fluent descent of the stairs and the agility with which I picked my way between the creaks in the floorboards to the kitchen.

– The kitchen at last!

I walked over to the door to the garden in order to test the weather and savoured deep draughts of air before slowly pushing the door shut. Once it was closed I felt more resilient and enjoyed the challenge of reaching for the tissues. As long as I floated particular actions on a tide of rhythmic movement, I averted their breakdown. The tissue was in the bin before I'd had a chance to register blowing my nose. This time I hadn't needed the usual six goes at trying to release the tissue from my fingers as I threw it at the bin.

I moved to the table where my glasses had been carefully positioned the previous night. With my hands behind my back I gauged the right distance to stand so that by leaning forward the wire arms of the glasses would glide neatly over the top of my beard without my having to use my hands.

'Idomeneo hum.' Swiftly my left arm swung from behind my back to lift and tuck the flexible curl of wire behind my left ear. My head began to sink into the patchwork cushion on which my glasses were resting.

– Just how tough is the toughened glass of the lenses? How much pressure can it take? Don't think about it – there's still the right-hand side to do!

I had two possible routes. Left hand over the top of the glasses to the right ear and adjust the wire; this was the more stringent test of my abilities. If that failed, I could fall back on the easier, lower route of under my beard and up the side of my chin. I decided to chance the upper route. I set out by crawling along the ledge of my eyebrows, taking great care to avoid touching the frame.

I tried to cross my forehead quickly before the tremor broke out and dislodged the glasses from the bridge of my nose and sent them crashing to the floor. My fingers met the resistance of sweaty skin. I overcame this with a final push. Wisely, I resisted the temptation to relax, and with a single sweep took hold of the wire and brought it to rest securely behind my right ear.

My head was still pressed into the cushion. Swinging my arm back behind me I slowly prised my face away and with the help of deep breaths swung upwards, standing still for a short while to savour the heightened clarity my vision had acquired.

Socks presented no problem, as for some time I had been in the habit of wearing the previous day's socks through the night and using them for running the following morning before discarding them into the wash. I had tried wearing my shoes in bed but it was just too uncomfortable and I worried that it might be bad for my feet. Some of my toe-nails had begun to die, though I suspected that this was the result of too little blood flow to the extremities because of my reduced blood pressure while I was taking the drugs.

I stooped down and slowly pulled each shoe into position below the chair ready for levering them on. Laces were left in a permanent knot, which naturally increased the difficulty of squeezing my feet in. I had tried shoe-horns without success, but then discovered that my monster porridge spoon was as effective in forcing on shoes as it was in stretching my mouth.

I got up, walked over to the drawer and bent to lift out the huge stainless-steel spoon. Wedging it between heel and shoe and pulling the flap up with my left hand while pushing down with my legs, I got the shoes on.

– Not bad going, that, I thought once I had managed to sit upright again.

– Yes but look at the door – the key's not in the lock!

As I rocked backwards and forwards to gain momentum to unstick myself from the chair, I felt a stiffness spreading with the emotional arousal caused by this set-back.

– What if I can't find the flippin' key? Why do we have to lock up anyway? Come off it – we've got to lock up for the insurance and everyone's agreed not to use the bolts.

I managed to stand up but was stuck in a curved bow with my fingers interlocked behind my back.

I must get calm. 'Idomeneo hum, idomeneo hum.' No good – something more elaborate was needed. I decided that the first thing to do was to stand straight. I unplugged my fingers from each other and immediately let my body keel over further, following my arms to the floor. As soon as the tips of my fingers touched the rush matting, the sensation was exaggerated into something like an electric shock which catapulted the top half of my body out of its curve.

Hands went up from my sides to my shoulder: side – shoulder, side – shoulder – then *whumph*, they snaked behind my back and two fingers of my left hand docked neatly into the palm of my right. I moved towards the cupboards.

'Idomeneo hum.' I positioned myself a couple of feet away and began falling rhythmically against the cupboard door, using outstretched arms to spring back each time. Fall forwards, 'Idomen one two . . .', push back, '. . . eo hum three four five'. Fall forwards, 'Idomen six seven . . .', push back, '. . . eo hum eight nine ten'. Fall forwards, 'Idomen one two . . .'

The stiffness melted away as my mind became filled with the nonsensical chant. I allowed myself to indulge in mild congratulation at having devised such a well-pitched strip of nonsense.

As if in answer to my prayer, the key appeared beneath an envelope I accidentally nudged; a wave of relaxation and relief flowed through my body. The drops of perspiration that were beginning to break out were magically dried and I felt warm. I took hold of the key, walked nimbly to the door, shoved it straight into the lock and, without any rattling, pressed with my thumb until the lock slid gently back. I pushed the handle down, eased open the door and drank in the fresh air once again.

To Grantchester

– Marvellous – I think there's a slight breeze starting up from the south-west.

I forced myself to forget the damp chill of my T-shirt left by my worry over finding the key.

– That will dry out in no time, but do I need my track-suit top?

– If you're going out to Grantchester you might start sweating while you're miles from home and that could be disastrous. Your arms will be covered and you may be unable to lose heat.

– But I'll be able to unzip the front.

– Yes, but that runs the risk of concentrating cooling on those body areas containing vital functions. Remember that article you read.

– Yes. What I need is a track suit with zips down the arms and sides as well as the front.

– Don't forget how your glasses get steamed up when you're too hot. You won't be able to see. Anyway, you even have trouble with the single zip on your track suit.

I began to go over the considerations again. How good a state was I in? How long was I going to be out for? Was I going to Grantchester? How favourable was the weather for helping maintain a balance of body temperature? How late had I left it? Were there likely to be many people about? It all boiled down to whether I could maintain a balance between heat generation and muscular fluency. The idea I had been considering was whether heat energy could compensate for the shortfall in resources for muscular control.

– I can't spend any longer going over all these things. I'm going to Grantchester and sod the track suit.

A moment later I was hurtling through the air, past my neighbour's car and twisting right into Pemberton Terrace. I gave the spring in my legs only fleeting attention. I didn't have to worry about whether I would be able to reach the cycle barrier on Brookside. My body sped through and, at the last moment, with inexplicable timing, my hands flew backwards like a braking parachute and grabbed hold of the iron-cold bollards.

Wrenched out of running, I stood tilting at the edge of the narrow pavement that borders the A10 London road. Relying mainly on sounds, I took a quick glance to confirm that the road was clear and let myself fall into the next stage. I paid little attention to the nimble-footed way my feet negotiated the kerbs.

– This is good and there's nobody about.

I reckoned the time was about five thirty. As I sneaked past the school on the left and the hotel on the right, both were fast asleep. The slight incline of the road propelled me forwards rather faster than I dared keep up for long.

Time to test the brakes and recover posture. I managed to stop within a very short distance. It was tempting to grasp hold of the lamp-post, but I wanted to practise braking without outside help in case aids were unavailable. Hands quickly behind my back, best foot forwards, now the right – and I was walking. The grinding drone of the bin lorry slowed me down.

– Good grief, they're early.

The noise was coming from deep within the cluster of school buildings; it disturbed me even though the men were unlikely to appear. I broke into a run and, crossing the hump of the bridge, sensed the stream of cooler air flowing along the river.

– That cyclist who's just gone past: I didn't care about him – or was it a woman? Oh, I must be on good form!

The causeway continued ahead as I careered left along a path bounded on either side by an expanse of green. Although I wasn't yet into open country, my relaxation was pushed a few degrees higher and a hint of the joy to come flickered over my skin. I began to hit patches of sunlight along the route. Without stopping, I risked a glance behind to see a vast area of blue sky with hardly any clouds. No one around. I slowed down and ran with my arms windmilling in a backwards butterfly stroke.

I pitched left again into Grantchester Road and on past the remaining houses. The road changed into a narrow lane, signalling a new domain. New sounds erupted. Birds porpoised along the hedgerows on either side. I couldn't believe they hadn't seen me and thought they must have been animated by my own playful mood.

I reminded myself to try harder this time and avoid the mistake of using the fluency humming through me for thinking. It was going to be a struggle because I had a lot of things on my mind, particularly ideas about the illness that were clamouring for clarification. How often I had arrived back home having spent the time figuring out solutions which were quickly lost beyond the barrier of my rapidly changing state of mind. So often I had wasted the enjoyment of the run and missed the harmony in which I flowed along, thoroughly merged into the surrounding scene.

– Grass, birds, hedge, sun, sky, river, leaves, blue, trees, corn . . .

The words of the countryside were thrown out loud as sheet anchors to hold back the drift into introspection and internal dialogue. If I lost myself too completely, however, there would be little to remember once back home. It would all be too easy, with few landmarks of progress and achievement. Maybe that is how it should be: the events of a journey remaining hazy and serving simply as the means for gaining a state of empty calm. But the mind's eye wants a role, noting sensations, subtly converting and organising them on the way.

The growing warmth from the sun away over the fields to my left called for my attention. My eyes locked into its brightness; a few moments of blindness. Mist still hung over the river.

– I wonder if I can reach it before it evaporates?

Intoxicated by the beauty of the scene, I stared too long and was caught. My running had carried me beyond the section of road I had unconsciously scrutinised for obstruction. I was on uncertain ground, running blind. My left foot struck something hard; I stumbled forwards, arms snaking up in protective anticipation of a fall. I'd strayed too near the edge of the road and my foot had dropped into a grid I had failed to see. The controlled falling by which I managed to run was now out of control: my legs stamped forwards at a faster and faster rate; my heart banged into panic gear; and my eyes reacted to the emergency by darting in all directions in search of something to grasp.

The self-fulfilling spiral was triggered. Awareness of probable danger heightens arousal, making it more difficult to cope because resources are wasted in worry. Reinforcements are then withheld to deal with the expected emergency.

– You've had it now. You're in for a heart attack.

– It's true my legs are giving way.

– It's miles back home.

– Shurrup.

– I'm beginning to sweat.

– Shurrup, shurrup. Idomeneo hum.

– What are you going to do when they find you stuck out here unable to get up?

– Stop it. Idomeneo hum. A tree!

– No it isn't.

– Must be a tree – with a branch.

My left hand jerked up and grabbed for the imagined branch. Grasp, stretch, straighten. My back stretched upright and balance was clawed back. Legs slowed and shuddered to a halt.

The tree had disappeared but its image had worked. My body keeled over and my outstretched hands rested on the ground in front of my toes.

– You can't stay like this. Get up.

I let myself drop a fraction more and, to the rhythm of my panting breath, I slowly uncoiled. To consolidate this victory of posture regained, I did my arm ritual until my hands were locked firmly together behind my back. It was tempting to launch off into the cooling space ahead.

– But I must check myself after a shock like that.

– Why bother? If you discover anything wrong it will only upset you and make it worse!

– No, it's too risky to ignore it. I must decide whether to go on or turn back.

It was so easy to convince myself I was coping when in fact larger and larger muscles were taking up the strain, risking complete collapse.

– Squeeze fingers. Good. No tremor in the legs and only slight rigidity. Swing arms up and touch your nose. Each in turn. Now both together. Fine. Muscles are holding out against the strain. Hands behind back again. Fall forwards. Run a few steps. Tilt backwards. Stop. Hold steady. Excellent.

Tests like this usually worked, although sometimes I was cruelly deceived into thinking muscles were more fluent than they really were. It takes careful checking to tell whether the maintenance or improvement in fluency is real or has been gained through the back being induced to take on the strain.

In an emergency, resources are released from higher-level storage. But there is no hope of storage at this general level being replenished until the next shot of cell activity, which seems to occur only twice every twenty-four hours, at about four in the morning and four in the afternoon.

– That's it, we're tuned to make available resources, either by producing or releasing already-produced chemicals to cope with the bombardment that starts once we're awake. And the timing is linked to sunrise and sunset.

– That *is* it! That explains why when Jan hasn't slept she's in a hopeless state until four in the afternoon when her mood changes and her face comes alive. It explains why I go running so early in the morning. But only partly, since there are social factors too.

– But the illness is supposed to mean that I haven't got any cells to be switched on or to produce the chemical storage for release at these two magical periods.

·– Well, the boost in fluency about four each morning corresponds closely with the amount of drugs I've taken the previous day. Part of the day's intake must still be swilling around when I go to bed and gets taken up by whatever cells remain. Then it's released at dawn the following day. So the illness leaves the rhythm mechanism undamaged.

– Remember the first few months of taking the drug? It was as if I was reliving my adolescent spurt!

– It's a hell of a fundamental chemical, then.

– Hey, this links up beautifully with dreaming!

I was doubled over, my hands touching the ground. Were my reflections simply a ploy to undermine the ambition to carry on the run by producing excitement over worthless ideas, or were these ideas a reflection of my heightened fluency? It didn't matter; I'd been seduced again and was in danger of getting stuck.

– Idomen one two eo hum three four five . . .

– I think there were some ideas there, but how to remember them. Dreams, sex, the sun, the drugs – they're all linked.

– Idomen . . . six seven . . .

– What's that?

There was a rolling sound of heavy tyres. My eyes strained to see through my steamed-up glasses. Anxiety flipped between fogged lenses and the approaching vehicle. How daft I'd been to risk sacrificing everything in the pursuit of ideas. The only way to clear the lenses was to get running and let the air do it. No question of my cleaning them. Anyway, I'd never get them back on.

I hung there suspended, as if waiting to be caned, peering intensely and hopelessly at the grey wall an inch ahead.

– No doubt about it – that's a handbrake.

By curling my head further between my legs I managed to see beyond the top of my glasses.

– Oh plod! It's a police car.

As they walked towards me I started to giggle. Two officers confronted by my upturned backside, laughter breaking out round my ankles. How would they react?

'Good morning, sir. Having problems are we?'

'No, I'm all right. I'll just get myself upright and then I'll explain.'

'That's all right, sir. Take your time.'

'It may take a few minutes, but please just wait.'

'That's all right. We've got plenty of time.'

'Thank you.'

I felt the blood throbbing through my head in a frantic search for something that would work. I pumped forwards images of calm: lying down listening to water trickling over stones close by; at sea, gently steering a boat, sails slowly flapping in a mild breeze.

– That's the one.

The boat rocked gently from side to side. I reached down for a bucket to draw some water from over the side, first stooping, then straightening.

– I'm up. Great.

I was ready to resume the conversation. The same officer spoke. 'Well done! Can we help in any way?'

I began to shake. 'No, I'm all right. Really.'

Would they feel offended by this rejection of help? Once before I'd got stuck and told a man who had crossed the road to help that I was very grateful but I could manage. Despite taking great care not to offend him, I heard him muttering abuse as he walked off.

'You seem a bit cold. You're shivering. Are you sure we can't take you home?'

'No, it's not shivering, it's shaking. I've got Parkinson's disease.'

My mind started to debate the relationship between shivering and shaking. Were they different or the same?

– Leave it for later.

Sensing that further delay would probably make me worse, the officer simply made a move back to the car, calling out: 'Cheerio, then,' and with his silent companion reversed back down the road.

Launched back into the run, I was pleased to be able to forget the incident and revive the sensations of the countryside. The fiery orange dish of the sun hung above tiers of trees, empty brown fields, long strips of yellow corn and fat wedges of green beset with placid cows. I listened to the slap of my shoes on the road and noted an unfamiliar bird call. It was easy to shut out the spoiling drone of traffic along the new motorway.

Joy returned with the running, and the running improved with my joy. On past a heap of manure, I twisted with the road as it dropped down towards a sharp right-hand bend. Elm logs were stacked for winter fires. I turned the next corner and passed the warming row of terraced cottages with their textured colours of hand-made brick.

Running Home

A slight incline meant that I was able to relax part of the effort of holding posture by tilting forwards a few more degrees without losing control. I approached the point where I left the road and began my return journey, crossing a field to join a footpath through the water-meadows. A few yards before the gate to the field I shuddered to a halt and stood still for a minute, swinging my arms behind my back and drawing myself sharply upright.

I started to feel a slight tension, first in my fingers, then wrists, arms, legs and on up to the muscles in my back. To combat this I imagined sluice-gates being forced open and water trickling out, then a series of waterwheels on a small stream beginning to turn, one after another, as the trickle became a flow.

I squeezed my fingers together, forced my arms straight and pushed my shoulders back. By stretching I imposed an increased load on my arms, shoulders and back; that set up a strain and a need to cope which induced stress. By removing the stress, a flood of resources became available for other muscles, in this case my legs.

– The level of storage seems fairly high still!

I checked round my body to make sure that the strain was not being translated into rigidity.

– No, very little rigidity.

I gave in to the temptation of speculation and the attendant risks of excitement.

– Acupuncture!

A friend had recently been to China to investigate acupuncture and had concluded that, although it did little to cure illness, it was successful in relieving pain. Surely acupuncture worked by imposing stress upon very localised points of the body and inducing a release of powerful painkilling chemicals – the opiates. Perhaps these facilitated neural transmission of the chemical I lacked.

The notion of meridians could be reinterpreted. The nervous system is not a fixed pattern of connecting pathways. Connections occur in the brain, where a network of stores form a web-like arrangement so that excessive demand made on one part reverberates through all the others and initiates a process of rescheduling the allocation of resources. Perhaps if the stimulation of a particular point increased demand above the availability of local storage, then the resources for other points would be released.

On one occasion in France, climbing a hill studded with thorn bushes, I got scratched to bits and experienced a remarkable increase in muscle fluency. Similarly, during the night when I am stuck, unable to move, the pressure from particular parts of the body gives me a pain-filled night, but curiously this is often followed by a day of considerable bounciness despite having had hardly any sleep.

– Maybe I should sleep on a bed of nails!

I heard the gate clank behind me and had to concentrate completely on avoiding the fresh cow splats. Foot co-ordination was tested to the limit as my body tilted nimbly to avoid each new threat. I enjoyed this game of dodge-and-weave. No stopping on this stretch; like a ballistic missile I must go single-mindedly for the target – that thin strip of grey path shaved out in the grass. The thick tufts were moist from yesterday's rain. Each quick step was gauged to avoid the damp penetrating my running shoes – my feet must be kept warm and dry.

– I'm nearly there!

My feet hit the hard surface. I stopped for a moment before shifting into a gentle trot after the charge across the field; the relaxation allowed me to experience joy as the solitary witness of the scene. I suddenly felt myself skipping and walking backwards to celebrate the playful springiness in my legs. Just at the point where I might have lost control, I flicked myself back round and marched on, swinging my arms extravagantly.

To my right green meadows stretched to the water's edge. It was tempting to leave the path in search of the sights and sounds of the river bank.

– Interesting: my sense of smell is keener. Why not take a look at the river?

Curbing such an ambitious idea, I made myself keep to the path. For me, as for Cinderella, the good times could last only so long. The gods kept a watchful eye out for such presumptuous disregard of the limitations decreed by my illness.

I was running again. A slight breeze cleared the haze from my glasses. My left hand reached up behind, two fingers gripped my T-shirt and the air was wafted up and down my back by wrist movements timed with the running.

– That looks like smoke!

Driven by the constant need to prepare for novel circumstances, I couldn't help wondering if this was a danger signal.

My run up to the gate was quite fast. I had forgotten to worry about the nettles on each side of the narrow path, but some careful dancing and manoeuvring got me through unstung and I burst out of the shade into the made-up road flanked by the houses of Newnham. I couldn't help the crunching noise of my feet on the road. Silly to bother about waking people, but I thought the milkman inconsiderate as he clattered his bottles in and out of the crates.

'Mornin'.' My confidence must be very high to be initiating this kind of social contact. He acknowledged my greeting. I had to believe he did, otherwise I risked a whole cloud-burst of thoughts to explain the rejection.

Along the stretch of unmade road, peace and quiet was restored. The nature reserve on the right was strangely silent. Maybe birds exhaust themselves with their territorial cries at the start of the day. Their quietness probably meant they were getting down to the serious business of finding food, just as I have to shut off as soon as I take on an important goal that requires concentration. It means substituting activity on a broad front for single-channel functioning and a narrow focus of attention.

My hands groped among the overhanging strands of leaves and gripped the posts on each side of the wooden stile. With perfect automatic judgement I raised my foot on to the step and heaved myself over the barrier, deftly shifting the strain from one arm to the other and one leg to the other. I quickly looked away from the clump of dog mess that lay in the path where I was about to tread.

– Don't let it get to you. Avoid anger at all costs. Look at that huge cobweb.

Amazingly swift movement of the spider. The fresh scents of the open countryside had given way to a dank heaviness of moisture-laden foliage and rotting wood. Nimbly side-stepping the slushy bits that lingered after the last downpour, and avoiding threatening branches by knitting the different moves into one continuous glide, I danced along the black path, deeper into the wood.

I singled out a smell from the coalescing vapours and an alarm sounded in my mind. It was the smoke I'd seen earlier. My brain speeded up and I felt my leg muscles tightening. The path forked; one way led down to the river's edge, the other curved more deeply into the wood; they merged again at the start of a field of tall grass. I took the second way to avoid the risk of meeting fishermen. My hearing, geared up to a high pitch, registered every sound. I could hear the crackling of burning wood. The safer route was now transformed into an unexpected threat. Voices . . .

– Young or old, rough or gentle, drunk or sober?

My resources were limited after the episode with the police. I didn't want to treat this as a full-blown emergency because my storage must have been considerably depleted. Temporary reallocation to my legs for flight could only be sustained for a short burst.

– Calm down. What the hell are you so worried about?

The smoke was all around me, captured in the net of intertwining branches. The wood came to an end a stone's throw ahead.

– Just ignore the smoke!

I heaved myself up on to a higher level of self-management and induced calm. I heard laughter and accelerated as fast as I dared as soon as the trees thinned, leaving me exposed.

– Two youths. No, three – there's one up on the branch overhanging the path.

I'd got to run under him. They'd set fire to a tree.

'Hey you!' one of them called.

– Oh, no!

More laughter . . .

'Hey you!'

– Keep going.

Tall grass on either side of me.

– Don't stop. Are they following? I must slow down.

My shoulders began to move upwards and backwards. Heavy feet banged life into the old wooden planks of a bridge across the drainage channel.

– I'll stop at the swing-gate at the end of this bridge.

The iron thwacked into my stomach as my hands failed to push it forward with sufficient speed. I rested, stooped over and holding on, panting.

As my mind caught up with the panic, my senses regurgitated memories of the experience. I uncurled and clasped my hands together behind me. My misted glasses signalled a rise in body temperature.

Maybe all kinds of arousal and emotion are developments of temperature regulation, I thought. When babies cry it often means they are too hot or too cold. The cry breaks out when a change takes body temperature outside the permitted range. Arousal and emotion arise through change, novelty, discrepancy and interruption.

Completely still, I tried to arrest the flow of sweat that had broken out. The mental effort was enormous, and failed.

– What if they had pushed me in the river? I could have swum downstream. No, I couldn't. I wouldn't have lasted two minutes in that freezing water. They might have tripped me up, making me career headlong against the burning stump. Don't be stupid. Yes they could. They wouldn't realise the problems I'd have. All it would take would be for my glasses to fall off to reduce me to helplessness. One of them had a knife. The one up the tree. Black leather jacket and Mohican hair-cut. He spat at me. Or had he just been spitting? Did he spit at me? I'm sure he did. Come off it, I went past them like a bullet. They probably ignored me completely. Then why did they call out? I don't know, forget it all anyway.

I felt the chill from the soaking T-shirt. A deadline imposed itself. I had to get home soon. If I wasted resources drying out the T-shirt I would probably lose muscular control. The wind would help, but my T-shirt was drenched. What I needed was one that worked like a nappy liner.

Stooped and running on my toes, I sped up the sloping steps of the iron bridge across the river. I didn't bother to check if the fishermen had arrived, but I heard the splash of an early-morning swimmer as he joined the ducks, some flying up in rage, others following his lazy strokes in the water.

– That guy in the tree really did have a knife!

I began the last gently rising stretch of the run. Faster past the anxiously muttering stream. Mist had evaporated from my glasses. If they had remained steamed up, I had decided to hide them somewhere and return later; cleaning them was out of the question. I had to run just fast enough for the air to clear them but not so fast that I got too hot and increased my rate of sweating.

Once out of the shade of the trees I could feel the sun's warmth striking my shoulders and chest, relaxing the muscles in my legs. I celebrated by jumping round and running backwards.

– Why worry? The sun is strong enough to dry your T-shirt.

Anticipating the moment when I might have fallen, out of control, I skipped round, stopped and turned to face the wall bordering the path. I wanted to stretch my arms before tackling the final part of the run.

I positioned myself a short distance away and fell forwards. Just in time to meet the contrived emergency, my arms sprang up to stop my face crashing into the wall. Elbows bent, my fingers and wrists flicked my body backwards off the wall. As soon as the rigidity in my arms had been relieved, and avoiding the temptation to see how many push-offs I could do, I swivelled round on the balls of my feet and ran to meet the fresh challenges of the A10.

It was about an hour and a half since I'd set out. Although it was still early, a steady stream of cars filled the road in both directions. Like Moses waiting for the waves to part, I searched for a gap in the traffic.

– No, relax and recover for another try. Yes.

I dashed forwards across the path of the half-asleep drivers, startled by this jolt to their slowly awakening metabolism. I didn't stop until I'd reached the top of the raised bank on the other side.

The way across Bateman Street was blocked by a solid row of cars waiting to turn on to the main road. Stuck there, I shifted the tremor from one leg to the other and, by dancing on the spot, made the strain endurable. I gripped my hands even tighter behind my back. Drivers and passengers, bored waiting in the queue, seemed to lock their gaze on me. I found myself grinning – or was it a grimace?

They moved at last and I was through the gap. I slowed to give another runner a chance to get ahead. He crossed by the pelican crossing. No use to me – the combination of deadline imposed by the lights and self-consciousness stirred up by the curiosity of stopped drivers had once reduced me to a snail's pace. Towards the end of that nightmare crossing I had broken into laughter.

– Perhaps laughter is another way of releasing tension, in the same way that tremor dissipates rigidity.

– Just concentrate on getting home!

At last, the end of my road. I'd refused to relax until this final stretch, but with the house in view, tension was replaced by carefree confidence. I toyed with the idea of going round the block, but I put aside this flippant adventure, turned left into St Eligius Place, skimmed along the side of the car, ducked under the washing line and reached the back door.

– Why doesn't Jan move the flaming line? Why don't I move it?

How was it that something so apparently critical as moving a neck-high washing line occurred to me when I was off the drugs, only to be completely forgotten when I had taken them and was able to do something about it?

The door clicked shut. Plonked down in a chair, I inevitably lost the race between keeping calm and pouring in sweat.

A Hard Day's Night

'Hello, how are you feeling?' my friend Steve greeted me.

'Bloody awful. Last night was dreadful.'

'What happened? Did you do too much yesterday?'

'No, not really. This just happens from time to time. Well, you might as well know – taking the drugs allows me to make love and last night, to make sure it worked smoothly, I took quite a lot. Then later I woke up unable to move. The sheet stuck to me and I got caught up in the blanket. I had to call Jan, which is something I hate doing. She came and changed me and the bed. I didn't wake until eight this morning. I felt awful and had to take the drugs.'

Jan is uneasy about love-making when I'm off the drugs. Apart from being generally out of control, my body becomes a dead weight. I remember seeing Jane Fonda in *Coming Home*, a film about a Vietnam war veteran who was confined to a wheelchair. They had an unorthodox, but nonetheless beautiful, way of making love. I took encouragement from this example and tried not to let the difficulties spoil things.

I had climbed out of Jan's bed with a warm feeling of joy, walked bouncily to my room and immediately fallen asleep. I had taken quite a lot of drugs unusually late in the evening; their effectiveness wore off at about two o'clock and I went zooming down to the depths of tremor and rigidity. I tried to change my position and found that I couldn't break the tremor. I was lying on my right shoulder; if I could get on to my back just for a short time it was likely that some control would return, but the tremor was so strong that I couldn't lift my left arm across my hip to lever myself over.

I began to worry and that made the tremor worse. Then I got hot and broke into a sweat. That really did worry me; it made it virtually impossible to move because the damp sheet stuck to me. So the crisis spiralled on, leaving me totally trapped like Agamemnon in his bath when Clytemnestra ensnared him in a net before stabbing him to death.

I was faced with two rotten alternatives. One was to stay soaking wet under the blanket and just lie there waiting for body heat to dry me out.

The other was to repeat nonsense to get as calm as possible and, by catching myself unawares, try to snatch the blanket over my body and roll on to the floor. I tried the second alternative. The awful thing was that I lost the momentum of the lurch and ended up stuck on the floor, cold and wet and not knowing what to do for the best.

I didn't really want to call Jan. She was due to start a new full-time job the following month and was trying to establish a pattern of sleep. The more often I called her in the night, the more lightly she slept as she held herself in readiness, anticipating my cries for help. But the cold meant I had to call her. The decision was a kind of signal to give up trying and I slowly sank from a kneeling position until my forehead was pressed into the carpet as if I were praying to Allah.

I called out, but my voice was too weak to break into Jan's sleep. I remembered a way of calling that had worked before once I got it going. This was to call Jan's name in quick succession, so that the series of weak cries produced an effect equivalent to one loud call.

'Jan, Jan, Jan, Jan, Jan, Jan . . .' It worked. I heard movement and was immediately filled with an odd mixture of relief and remorse.

'I'm sorry, Jan,' I mumbled into the carpet, listening intently for her reassurance that it was all right. But Jan was dazed and confused. What a bloody contrast: strength and smooth fluency had so quickly been replaced by total collapse and weakness.

'Try to bounce me up, Jan. Don't risk putting your back out.'

She took both my hands and, using her own body as a counter-weight, raised me part of the way, lowered me back down again and then leant back and pulled until I was standing up.

'I'm sorry, Jan, but could you change the sheet and the pillow-case, and get me a dry T-shirt and track-suit bottom? But first could you help me do a wee?'

Jan could hardly hear my whispering and was probably too sleepy to follow my series of requests. She knew what to do anyway. She tugged off the T-shirt, which was clinging tightly to my damp body, reached for the towel behind the door and rubbed me down. Then she pulled down my track suit and slowly frog-marched me to the basin. The cold-water tap was turned on to wash away the surge that started as soon as I stood with my hands clasped behind my back. Luckily the basin was just the right height!

'Never mind, Ive. Don't worry.'

A cloud of misery immediately lifted. Jan now got on with changing the sweat-soaked sheet and doing the other things in an efficient businesslike way.

'Anything else?'

'No, that's fine. Thanks very much indeed – and I'm sorry.'

I lay there quite still and heard the click of the door as she returned to her bed. But soon I felt the need to change my position. I began to move my right leg and then I noticed that the blanket was damp against my bare arm.

'Sod it. Why hasn't she changed the blanket?'

I pushed back my growing irritation and resentment. Throughout the illness I have had to fight constantly the tendency to find a scapegoat to blame each time difficulties arise. It is a continual struggle to prevent unreasonable and pessimistic thoughts from taking over.

It was now half-past three and I lay there waiting for the curious phenomenon of the early-morning boost of renewed fluency to work its magic once again. It was no good trying to get back to sleep. The crisis had triggered a release of coping resources so that my wakefulness would last for a few hours at least.

Interruptions didn't always arouse me to a state of full attention. Usually I could cope with the noisy return of Justin or Sophie in the early hours, with the strain of rigid muscles becoming painful, or with feeling too hot or too cold, provided I could avoid thinking about the disturbance. In a similar way, if I could change position or move the bedclothes without having to use elaborate strategies or tactical manoeuvres, I might escape being cheated of getting back to sleep.

This time, though, things had gone miles too far. The combination of my whole body being wet, cool air wafting from the open window, the anxiety of having to wake Jan and the feeling of bleak sadness at my failure to cope on my own had released a rich cocktail of chemicals in my brain. It had all happened too early and by the time it was light, about five o'clock, much of my early-morning fluency would have been wasted. Instead of the gentle flowing through my limbs that I had come to expect each morning, fluency had been forced upon me. I decided not to get up but to try instead to think through what had been happening. I would sacrifice some of the resources for my run to try to develop some sort of model to help unravel the complexity.

Images began to flow through my mind. A waterfall with ledges of rock interrupting its descent and dividing its single flood into numerous subsidiary falls; then each of these struck rocks which broke up the cascade even further. This suggested some sort of hierarchical arrangement, but failed to encompass the notion of storage that I was beginning to develop.

Running back from Grantchester one morning I had seen an exceptionally vivid sunrise. Dawn had erupted across the eastern sky in crimson ribbons, threading their way from the sun through light wisps of cloud. This was a better analogy than the waterfall, as it incorporated the idea of a source of energy, the sun, feeding along channels with interim points of storage, the clouds. But why not a number of separate sources? And were the paths related to each other hierarchically or did they form a network?

The image of the sun was a good one. Maybe its warmth triggered my increased fluency in the mornings. Perhaps sun worshippers had something after all. If I were ever to develop a need to seek comfort through allegiance to an external deity, then sun worship would be a serious candidate!

'What a business last night was – but it was lovely,' I thought. Love-making was one of the bonuses of the drugs, and I thought that if ever I lost that joy it might be the one thing to send me into depression.

Freud and Libido

I wanted to be sure that the degree of my disability could not be disputed in the future following the amazing improvements I was hoping to achieve, so I decided to make a video. The technician at college generously gave up his time to set up two cameras and other equipment. A friend drove me in to do the filming because I had deliberately stayed off L-dopa for three days to deplete storage and uncover a deep level of deficit. I had to be helped out of the car and fell along the corridors into the studio.

My aim was twofold: to record in vivid detail the full extent of the problem; and to show the strategies and tactics I had developed to get round the difficulties of everyday tasks such as dressing, taking off my jacket, getting up from a chair, writing, tying my shoe-laces and so on. I was pleased with the clarity of the recording and used it to illustrate two talks I gave in different departments of the university. On each occasion I offered to be available should anybody be interested in conducting research. I was disappointed by the lack of response.

I was obviously not going to make any progress in finding someone to use my ideas for research (apart from Professor Marsden's willingness to incorporate me into the work of his team) without publicity. So I sent the video off to the producer of the television documentary series *Forty Minutes*. He wrote back saying that he had watched it, had been deeply moved, but that unfortunately he didn't feel that he could use it. I was tempted to write back and tell him that he had got it completely wrong. My intention was not to move people, but to inform them in a matter-of-fact way about the features of Parkinson's. However, I simply let that one go.

Soon afterwards an article by Oliver Gillie appeared in the *Sunday Times*, reviewing the evidence concerning Freud's early experiences with cocaine. Gillie argued that there was no support for Freud's belief that one day a chemical would be found which would serve as the energy source of libido and sex. He wrote, 'The libido – the energy which fuels the machinery of Freudian psychology – remains in essence a mythical substance, akin to the fabled love potions'.

I was very excited; immediately I sat down and wrote a paper based upon my experiences of dopamine which I put forward as a strong candidate for the role of libido. I proposed that, rather than a hierarchical arrangement with sex at the top, insinuating itself into functions at other levels, it was more appropriate to think in terms of a network of functions of which sex was a component.

I discussed the paper at length with my sister Anne, who had read most of Freud's work and was a keen follower of his views. I kept talking about problems arising because energy got used up and the producing cells became exhausted; she put forward Freud's view that problems arose when opportunity to use energy became blocked.

Gillie's article described Freud's notion of 'noxae', which resulted from frustration caused by incompletion of action or non-resolution of conflict. These harmful substances were supposed to be produced in the brain when energy was available but could find no channel down which to flow.

This could be linked up well with a possible model based on stress in relation to the cause of Parkinson's disease. In situations of extreme sustained stress the brain could produce an outpouring of dopamine far in excess of the amount that could be used. The surplus chemical was then oxidised or broken down into simpler elements. The theory suggested that these oxidised chemicals or the process of oxidation might lead to poisoning of the dopamine-producing cells.

It is as if the brain were operating like a boiler with a broken thermostat. The boiler pumps out heat, but instead of the thermostat switching off the fuel supply to prevent overheating, it sends a message to produce more heat the hotter the boiler gets, until there is a catastrophic explosion. In some situations the brain might produce transmitters to cope with stress, but instead of controlling the situation the transmitters are used as an opportunity to take on higher levels of arousal. The brain then produces more and more transmitters until disastrous damage to dopamine-producing cells results.

Freud may have been wrong in identifying libido with sex. The flow of transmitters might be at its most intense during sex, but libido, or 'energy', seems to underpin a host of functions without reference to sex.

I was greatly influenced by my experience with sex, on and off my drugs. Off the drugs, sex was at the expense of the energy required for holding my muscles under control. If storage was depleted, sex would leave me in a far worse state than I'd been in before. If there was some storage available, sex would quickly exhaust it. I might be all right for a short while, but would deteriorate quickly as the debilitated cells proved incapable of maintaining production. For me, it was a question of conserving energy rather than of finding the means for its expression.

Psychoanalysis is of limited benefit because it assumes that rational awareness of troublesome memories is sufficient to neutralise their effect. The problem may be related to the levels of neural transmitters available when these memories are re-run in dreaming.

I suggested that creativity is the manipulation of transmitters by the temporary dampening of feedforward to allow feedback, followed by a boost to feedforward to impose a concluding structure on the new experience. Analysis and structuring are suspended temporarily to allow an uncritical, almost playful state, until a new pattern snaps forward into consciousness. It is analogous to the fairground waltzer in which you press the brake, then let go and spin forwards much faster.

Transmitters are also the key to the 'flow' experience of meditation and religious ecstasy. Meditation works by turning on cells to produce more transmitter or by inducing concentration of transmitter flow by reducing antagonistic emotion.

Dopamine and related transmitters serve as the means of coping. They are essentially the resource for feedforward readiness as opposed to feedback from outside events or internal concerns. They provide energy for both muscular and mental processes.

Gillie returned my paper and, although I had sent it to him without any thought of publication, he suggested that I submit it to *New Scientist*. They too found it interesting but suggested that I try another magazine less demanding of scientific credibility. I gave up, although I nearly persuaded Gillie to come to stay for a weekend with a view to writing an article about Parkinson's; but in the end he couldn't find the time. Once again I had to swallow my disappointment and look for another way forward.

Closely Observed Parkinson's

A friend, John Styles, offered to help me get my thoughts about Parkinson's down on paper. We had been having a drink together, discussing various ideas about the illness and about the effects of the drugs on my capacity and quality of thought. He had been very interested in what I said and I felt he would be a useful critic as he was not only a physicist but also accomplished in philosophy and computing. He had helped clarify my understanding of computers and had liked an idea that I had for a test of computer intelligence. I suggested that the task of editing one of my papers to produce two different versions – one for general readers and the other for people with knowledge of psychology or medicine – would be a good trick for a computer! We also toyed with the idea of writing a book together. Even if that didn't materialise, he would keep me on my mettle and help me avoid spouting nonsense.

I wanted to take a large dose of drugs before we started in order to create the most favourable state for speculation and fluency. It would also be interesting to see how the drugs affected my delivery and intelligibility. We decided to record on tape and transcribe later, as this would allow the ideas to flow freely without interruption.

I had been using the concept of 'energy' to describe the effects of dopamine and John added to my doubts about its appropriateness by insisting I define my understanding of the term. I certainly used it in a different way from heat energy, but wondered if chemical energy encompassed the role of neural transmitters. I had used the word 'resource' in my papers to Professor Marsden, but felt that 'energy' better described what I wanted to convey.

We had four taping sessions in all, at each one playing it by ear as to how far John would question me or leave me to blurt whatever I considered worth saying. We were both surprised when I spoke non-stop for three hours, with John intervening only briefly. The hours just seemed to vanish in no time. During one of the later sessions I careered ahead with my ideas and at the end asked John what he thought. He listed a number of topics that had intrigued him and I was surprised at the accuracy of his comments: he had been asleep for the last hour!

The transcription showed quite clearly that I'd been talking in a highly speculative way, making connections and creating syntheses, some of which later seemed plausible and others which were definitely not.

The two main threads running through the sessions were, first, the idea that dopamine can be considered a form of energy that can be managed, stored, conserved, channelled or wasted and, second, that the impact of emotion and arousal make the management of this energy so much more difficult for someone with Parkinson's.

At one stage I set out to discuss variations in the levels of energy required for action and thought. Once I was launched into the central theme, there was no limit to the number of ideas that I tacked on in subordinate clauses, ever increasing in their complexity. Looking over the transcript later on, we were surprised at the drugs' influence in producing a page-long sentence!

What one now does with the store of energy that one has built up is either successfully cope with a much greater variety of elements simultaneously than one otherwise was able to do or the energy may scour past experience which has been laid down in memory with a particular problem being held in a sort of position of context to which the rememberings are all related for the possibility of relevance and that the energy that one has stored allows this to recur and novel solutions to arise, the problem so often being that after this energy has flooded through one might have an experience of clarity and awareness of a solution, but when one returns to a prior level of energy flow that state is not conducive for remembering and being able to recall the clarity, the nature of the clarity, the nature of the solution that one achieved, but often it is successfully translated from one energy level into let's say the rational level of energy functioning and it's then recorded and it survives the experience itself for other people to try to appreciate either in the form of testing it out which is a scientific insight, or in terms, that is to say, of rational procedures which don't entail any extraordinary states of personal energy levels to be attained, or it may require, it may be wrapped up in metaphor in an indirect expression of what it was about and require the audience, the person who is now faced with this insight that has been communicated through this indirect metaphor by the person who experienced it – the whole realm of aesthetics comes in here – and the person, the metaphorical presentation, has almost, if it is to succeed, has almost got to induce momentary raising in the audience of their concentration

so that they will be able to appreciate by their own personal concentrated boost of energy focused upon what is before them, that is,
the presentation induces this concentration with a view to their
appreciating some of the insight for themselves which resulted in the
production that is before them; in other words, there is an experience
by an individual which is translated into some public form which in
turn has to induce back in the audience some sort of, some degree of,
some aspect of the original experience, so that if one's walking down an
art gallery looking at pictures it's not very conducive to the appreciation of those pictures to have a glass of wine in one hand and be
talking to a number of people because it does ideally require calm, that
is to say, calm which will cut out from consciousness concerns about
how one is sounding when one's talking to other people, how one
appears, who's looking at whom, who knows whom and so on, and also
calm in the sense of the production perhaps of further energy and one
is drawn to try to achieve this greater energy by a feeling of trust that
there's something in what is presented in the environment with the
potential for being shared and appreciated which brings up the notion,
the fundamental notion of love which is central to so much of human
interaction in existence and so on.

Through a friend I met Jon Alpert, who was over here from Yale
University conducting research on the part of the brain that was affected
in Parkinson's. It was through his efforts that one of the meetings at
which I had a chance to talk about my illness and illustrate it with the
video was held. Subsequently he offered to come round to my home and
help me record my observations.

I was very happy to have at last found someone willing to spend time
exploring and documenting the weird and wonderful features of Parkinson's disease. Jon's manner was ideal. During my frequent pauses he
would keep his gaze turned away, patiently waiting for the starter motor
of my speech to work. He stayed for a couple of hours at a time making
handwritten notes.

After a few sessions, Jon wrote to the editor of a journal to ask for
guidance about the sort of thing that might be acceptable for publication.
We received an encouraging response to the extract we sent in and I then
decided that it would be a good idea to separate my description of
situations from my theoretical discussion of broad themes.

On that basis, we built up a number of accounts of activities such as
running, cycling, making toast, sleeping, throwing a ball against a wall or
getting out of a chair, and a week or two later Jon arrived with a typed

draft. I squirmed among the piled cushions of my chair in an effort to get comfortable and quell my excitement, while he read aloud from the paper. After he'd left, I read it through: some of it was quite good!

When I am stuck in a cycle of tremor, I sometimes let the tremor go faster in order to override it and graft on a degree of voluntary control. By allowing it full expression I am able to lose it. It is as if one has exhausted and dissipated the forces driving the tremor or mobilised forces to put on the brakes.

I am frequently able to initiate voluntary movements despite the tremor. The main components of the action have to be free of tremor, though. The tremor has to be shifted elsewhere. I don't lose the tremor; I redistribute it to muscles not implicated in the immediate act.

Tremor is a mixed curse. Some acts appear to draw on the tremor before it disappears and to harness the energy for their own devices. It is as if they can gain from swimming with the current rather than against it.

When I hold back tremor intentionally, when I constrain it by an act of will, rigidity increases. However, I can sometimes lose tremor without the cost of rigidity in acts free of emotional attachment, such as grabbing the sides of my wing-chair. Indeed, tremor may even abate at the prospect that help is on the way.

Tremor, rigidity and slowness of movement seem so interrelated to me. I often think of them as strategies for expressing the same underlying defect. In different people tremor will exceed rigidity or stooped posture.

Tremor is particularly vigorous when arousal is high and there is a heightened readiness for action. Given a poor night's sleep, or if I have used up resources in drying myself with body heat, then instead of tremor a bland rigidity and immobility set in.

Quite often, much to the annoyance of people who are with me, the more helpless I become, the more I giggle and laugh. It may be a counter-reaction to the gloom around me. People tend to get fed up, as if blaming me for getting into such a helpless state. Possibly I use laughter as a tension release, to dissipate the stress that arises in the face of utter incapacity.

Sometimes, when I take the drugs, I get an immediate reduction in tremor; perhaps as in anticipation of relief by the cavalry coming. Shortly after, however, I sense increased heart rate. All sorts of problems crowd my consciousness. Content then contributes to arousal and further arousal generates new content. Another vicious circle!

I find that the drugs can be encouraged to 'take' by adopting a position with my knees apart, feet twisted outwards and my upturned hands resting on the arms of my chair.

One of the most striking things about taking the drugs seems to be the imperative that L-dopa be synthesised to dopamine, whether required or not.

Often I could enjoy a good metaphysical session with high intellectual fluency despite the tremor and lack of motor control. After taking the drug there is a slip back and a reduction in intellectual prowess as motor control is re-established.

When I get muscular fluency, I lose my inclination to carry out the plans I had before control was achieved. I have a greater capability of completing an act, but feel less inclined to undertake it. It is as if the planning function gets dried up and one is in a slightly depressed state. So I adopt strategies that take into account this shift and the delay in initiating action.

There seems to be a difference between relying on what I think of as storage and of using fresh exogenous dopamine. L-dopa produces a wonky person, a twisted person. I feel as if I can never relax.

When on the drug I succeed, but unlawfully. There is a sense of discomfort in my activities, almost as if there is latent dyskinesia, felt but unseen. If I am running, there is the impression of holding out until the run is completed rather than falling in with the activity. On the other hand, to go running in the early morning before I take the drugs, by drawing on storage, is marvellous, even with a degree of tremor.

Moderate tremor is quite relaxing really. It's as if, when I am in a state of controlled tremor on L-dopa there is a much more immediate and taut distribution of resources: a circuit which hasn't got an earth; a pressure cooker without an escape valve.

In making advances in my understanding, it is better to read when I am off the drugs. I am then in a state of openness. Ideas will flow over me and through me. Stimuli bombard me more directly. I will be more readily susceptible to shock and will be overwhelmed more readily. I find it difficult to put up physical or intellectual resistance. Before I began taking the drugs, I would start crying at the cinema.

In contrast, on the drugs there is a lurching and grabbing. I don't see any problems. It is akin to madness and ecstasy. 'Ecstatic' means standing outside, and that is how one feels.

After the first few months of taking the drugs my body showed signs of dyskinesia or writhing. Arousal, excitement and embarrassment exacerbate the writhing. I take my lunch on my own in college to avoid the effort of coping with people's attention.

From time to time I went to the Maudsley Hospital on a voluntary basis to take part in whatever investigations Professor Marsden's research team was conducting. On one occasion

I noticed a woman with intense dyskinetic movements and found myself responding with unusually profound writhing even on moderate doses of the drug. The experience seemed to give my body the excuse to release the symptoms.

My impression is that dyskinesia arises not simply from overproduction of dopamine which then bombards supersensitive receptors, but from fatigue and overloading. Something seems to have worked harder than it should have. I sense a withdrawal of control from my lips and I splutter.

A key factor in dyskinesia is whether there has been an intervening sleep between doses of the drug. Rest and sleep between doses augments motor control without increasing dyskinesia. In contrast, three doses without a rest in between can be disastrous.

It often appears that my failure to execute a movement is due to interference from the emotion aroused by the intention to act. So I have developed strategies for deceiving my body. When skipping I begin backwards and then switch to skipping forwards.

Modulation or redirection of an action also causes breakdown. So I establish highly predictable patterns which are unlikely to be interrupted in mid-course. In going to the post office, for example, I try to ensure I can manage the trip in one single lurch without interruption.

Once stopped in midstream I cannot get restarted. The momentum collapses and I must start again from the beginning. My motto has become: 'He who hesitates is lost; he who is interrupted is lost; he who is disrupted is lost.'

On the Loo

It was seven thirty on a Sunday morning. I'd been for a run, had a shower, successfully got part of my breakfast and had decided to take a chance with the loo. Each day I try to delay taking the drugs for as long as possible. However, there is a dilemma: I usually need to have taken them in order to go to the loo, which I may feel like doing soon after I get up. So I have a choice between trying but failing after considerable time and effort, or taking the drugs long before I want to.

I wasn't in too bad a state that particular morning and had a reasonable amount of storage laid down from the previous day's medication. My hands and arms shook but my legs were under control. I dropped my track-suit pants, plonked down on the seat, and drew my feet back until I was nearly on tiptoe. By swinging my arms I brought my elbows to rest on my knees and jammed my fists under my jaw with the knuckles of my index fingers lodged behind each ear-lobe. From there I nudged my fists slowly behind my neck, bending my head forwards until the fingers of one hand made contact with the other. I pushed my neck still further forwards, intertwining my fingers more tightly. By now the urge to go had gone!

– I wish Jan had agreed to my original plan. We could have had a special loo put in as well as the shower when we got the grant from the council. I could have got one of those pans where you squat right down, with bars to hold on to. It would have worked much better than this daft sitting position.

Once again I was distorting reality to provide myself with someone to blame for my predicament.

I knew I needed to go because I hadn't managed it yesterday, but I couldn't energise my bowels. I carried out a trial run to alert both muscles and brain to the imminent effort. I tightened the grip of my fingers, pulling my neck and head down towards my knees. I pressed with my feet against the floor so that my leg muscles took up most of the strain. Then my body began to shudder like a plane aborting its take-off run.

With difficulty I wrenched my fingers apart, turned my hands palms upwards and rested them on my knees. The mantric nonsense took over in an attempt to release resources to where they were needed. But I remained stuck. It was a little like not quite being able to recall a name that you know is there in your memory.

I focused on my immediate situation and tried to climb back into the empty world of my mantra. But the temptation to speculate was too strong. After all, didn't creative thought involve making insightful connections between apparently disparate ideas?

– Yes, but there are differences. You're stuck here unable to call upon resources, and creative ideas present themselves of their own accord. No: it may seem like that but often a huge effort has gone into considering a paradox or contradiction subconsciously. While I happen to be in a calm state doing something trivial, the induction process has been quietly mustering the means for coming up with an answer. That's not all that different. It's the difference in the lengths I have to go to to marshal adequate resources to make the creative leap, by sacrificing control over muscles not involved in the immediate task of pushing. What I have to do is let go of control. Yes, that's similar to the creativity of dreaming . . .

Having once opened the channel to speculation, it was difficult to divert the flow back to the immediate problem of 'straining at stools'.

– That's a daft way of describing it. Why not talk about trying to crap? It's as if you're trying to confer medical status by changing the language with which you think.

Like a teacher in a noisy classroom trying to quieten the chaos, I had nothing to fall back on.

– Oh yes, the mantra. I think I'd better try something else.

I looked at the window. A cold wind was blowing outside. I jerked it slightly open, sufficient to let the cool draught register as 'change' in the centre that regulates body temperature. It was a way of stressing the body into releasing resources it would otherwise hold back. A lot depended upon there being some still available, and if this didn't work I was going to give up.

As the cold air rushed down my uncovered legs I regained my position, gave a token push to register the priority and struggled to awaken the mantra to block off the channel to ideas. There was some movement in my bowels. I began to imagine the stored resources lined up like parachutists ready to be pushed out of the plane by the instructor.

– Hold it! Steady, steady, steady. Now!

I held back my breath and pushed with all my strength.

– Keep going!

At first things seemed to be going well, but then gradually tremor began to break out and odd words, each one a cryptic clue to rich reflection, forced their way past my more and more frantic muttering. It was becoming impossible to hold my breath any longer.

– Try panting – short, quick pants like they tell women to do when giving birth. Anaerobic and aerobic shift? Forget it! Concentrate!

Tap, tap, tap, tap. Thud, thud.

– You're going to wake everybody up! It's hopeless. Have a rest, just a short one, and then start again. No! If I stop now I'll never start up again. Think of the reward, the good feeling after such effort. No, stop thinking altogether.

Whether through stress or relaxation it all came to the same thing: banking up a wave of resource to explode forward.

– A total disaster!

I gave up and sat there staring into space. I was fairly calm, but exhausted. Shutting the window was easy, but I couldn't move to stand up. I must have waited at least five minutes. Eventually I decided I'd wasted enough time. I raised my arms above my head and as they were dropping down to my side I lurched to my feet with a plastic ripping sound!

I stood still and suddenly sensed contractions in my bowel. I imagined boulders tumbling down a dried-up riverbed. Hardly thinking what I was doing, I dropped my pants, sat on the seat, locked my hands behind my neck, took a massive deep breath. The landslide slowed.

– Quick before the wave subsides!

The sounds of success! I struggled not to notice, not to think about it, and tried to let it just happen. It was a race against time.

– Time, effort – how much achievement is crammed into the time?

I'd blown it again and would have to be satisfied with half an achievement. I sat on the bidet and turned on the hot and cold taps. I misjudged the mix and a boiling hot jet of water shot up against my skin. My mind leapt a mile; my body shifted a few inches and I dropped back. I managed to cut the flow and then turn down the hot tap. The pleasant sensuality of the spray allowed me to drift.

I imagined a clock face with labels of various concepts.

– 'Activity', 'Arousal', 'Coping', 'Attending', 'Thinking'. There's no set sequence. You can start at any point and move to any other point to suit different trains of thought. Activity may be induced to match arousal, or arousal may be induced by activity. Each function can assume a dominant role and use the other functions as explanatory variables. The direction of influence can be reversed. Ability to make such changes depends upon the tentativeness with which the ideas are held, the complexity of the network and the person's emotional commitment to the model.

– To appreciate new ideas you have got to slow them down and, at an extreme level, use meditation to look at individual frames of experience separately, like moving a film forwards frame by frame. In this way you get a chance to examine the detail afresh and playfully make new connections with other elements of experience.

– Ah! Someone must have turned on the hot tap in the kitchen!

The balance between hot and cold water had been lost and I began the slow process of standing up.

Part Three

Meeting Jonathan Miller

One day in March 1984 I reached for the morning's post and found a letter from London NW1. It took me a few moments to realise who it was from. Six months before, frustrated by my failure to get my study of Parkinson's off the ground, I had hit on the idea of contacting Jonathan Miller. I'd read somewhere that he had put aside opera and the arts to revive his earlier commitment to medicine.

The first letter I sent to him came back because the address was wrong. I have no idea why I didn't just give up, but Sue, my occasional secretary, made a special effort to find his current address and phone number by writing to his agent. When after a few weeks I hadn't had an answer to my second letter, I closed off that avenue of hope.

It was four months later that a reply came with an apology for the long delay; he had been in Canada keeping abreast of new developments in neurology. He said he would be very interested to talk to me and would like me to ring him, but not for a month or so because he was very busy. I waited for a month and then telephoned.

We spoke briefly and I got the impression that my performance was letting me down. Jonathan said later that he had tried to resist my faint, rather demanding voice insisting that he would find it profitable to talk to me. He promised he would write to me. Two weeks later I wrote him another letter, urging him all over again to come to Cambridge, even if only for a couple of hours. I would pay his fare and a fee for his time.

Now this letter from him had arrived. It suggested that I ring him on Friday night to confirm his intention of coming up the following day.

I was so grateful to Jon Alpert for all his help that I wanted him to share this occasion. He came round at ten o'clock on the Saturday, Jonathan Miller being due at eleven. We wondered if Jonathan would mind the microphone and tape-recorder we had rigged up. I was in a pretty shaky state: I had taken no drugs because I wanted not only to describe the illness but also to demonstrate it as fully as possible.

Suddenly the gate banged and I began my shaky journey to the door. The excitement was causing me to keel over, and by the time I had pulled the door open, my head was straining to look up rather than tip to the ground. Jonathan Miller and I exchanged hellos and I backed into the room, inviting him to follow me. I asked if he minded me calling him Jonathan. The contrast between our speech was enormous: he had a rich, deep, melodious voice, whereas I spoke in a dry whispering monotone. We sat down; his warm expression was reinforced by gentle concern and genuine interest radiating from his dark, hooded eyes. Soon we were deep in conversation and his whole body was alive with a harmony of gesture. I meanwhile alternately trembled out of control or locked myself into aching rigidity.

Soon I felt that I was winning and had captured his imagination. He was enthusiastic about the things I demonstrated and about my ideas. After an hour I was sufficiently confident to ask Jonathan if he was going to be able to stay for the afternoon. A hint of caution coloured the beginning of his reply as he said, 'There is somebody I have to see . . . but there's no fixed time for that.' It was in the bag!

I suggested we go into the garden.

'All right,' he replied, intrigued.

'I often come into the garden to throw a ball against this wall. It's surface is moderately even so that the way the ball returns is fairly predictable.'

'Yes, I see.'

'I can usually catch the ball with one hand. If I let the ball bounce on this rough ground first . . .'

'And it hits a bump . . .'

'That's exactly it! If it does, and goes in an unpredictable direction, I'm in trouble. Watch!' I pushed rather than threw the ball against the wall and caught it three or four times in succession. Then I let it bounce first; it hit a bump in the grass and went off at a different angle.

'Ah yes!' he exclaimed. 'You are unable to make the postural adjustment to reach it.'

'Yes. The key thing seems to be whether the ball arrives in arm's reach without requiring me to move my body. Now just watch what happens to the tremor as I use this arm to throw – watch my other arm and hand!' I carried out a series of throws and, as the tremor momentarily departed from muscles taking part in the movement, sure enough the control over non-participating muscles broke down.

'Did you see it?'

'Yes, I did. I suppose this is the rescheduling you were talking about. Now what I want to know, Ivan, is did you do that consciously or did it just happen?'

'I'm not sure; maybe it can be both, depending on how difficult the task is or how much control I've got. Let me show you this. If I bounce the ball and catch it, tremor disappears in the hand that does the catching. I'm puzzled by the way they distinguish between different kinds of tremor. There is tremor when I simply hold the ball without any intention of doing anything with it. Then if I think of an intention, the tremor increases.'

'Yes. Let's go inside and we'll talk about it.'

I was a bit taken aback – then realised it had been pouring with rain for the past five minutes!

Jonathan stayed over lunch, which for him consisted of a cup of coffee and a Mars bar. We continued our conversation and I took my drugs in order to show him what I was like in a state of control. I was very keen to demonstrate how successful I was in managing the drug-taking by myself, so I didn't want to take too many and end up writhing. On the other hand, he was bound to want to go soon and the drugs might not take in time. This made me anxious and, not surprisingly, delayed the drugs working. I felt sad as he got up to leave, but as he was putting on his lumpy brown coat and I had given up all hope of gaining control, the fluency began to rush through me and I could now demonstrate the contrast.

As he went off to meet the Master of his old college, Trinity, some of what he had said reverberated in my mind: 'We'll have to have a "recky". You're gold-dust to the TV trade. I think the best thing would be to make a film. Maybe I could come up one day a week within the remit of my research grant.'

Returning to the sitting room, I slumped into my chair, exhausted and elated at the same time. I allowed my thoughts to race ahead with all sorts of possibilities. Eventually I began to consider practicalities.

A week or two earlier I had thought that I might be able to give up work altogether and devote all my time to research into Parkinson's disease. In that frame of mind I had precipitously written to Professor Marsden telling him of my plans and hopes and asking him if he would be interested in my doing long-term research under his direction. He wrote back within the week suggesting that we should get together to discuss what and how! I felt embarrassed at the warmth of this positive response since I soon realised I could afford to give up work for only one term a year and, besides, there was now no knowing what might develop from Jonathan Miller's visit.

It was a case of everything beginning to work at the same time, with the resulting conflicts and incompatibilities between different avenues. I might be forced to choose between taking part in hard scientific research and some less rigorous endeavour which might nevertheless give greater publicity to my ideas. The last thing I wanted was to exhaust Professor Marsden's patience by getting him interested in a proposal and then dropping it. I hoped that he would understand. I wrote explaining that I had miscalculated about packing in my job altogether and offered to go to his unit for a couple of weeks in the autumn on the same basis as before. No reaction to my letter was needed: he would simply wait for me to contact him nearer the time when I was available.

Soon afterwards Jonathan telephoned to say that *Horizon* had agreed to make a programme with me.

Making the Film

I knew what I wanted to be put into the programme. I would use situations from real life to demonstrate ways of manipulating the symptoms. Jonathan and I would discuss each sequence and, finally, one or two experts, ideally including Professor Marsden, would join me and Jonathan in a panel discussion.

I was delighted that it would be a *Horizon* programme because that meant there would be at least fifty minutes; then I became greedy and wanted to know if it could go on for ninety minutes. The producer, Patrick Uden, said that it was fairly rare for them to go beyond an hour, but he would wait to see how the filming went and then decide whether to approach *Horizon*'s editor for a longer slot. There was so much I wanted to get across and I pinned my hopes on the longer time. I knew that if I didn't get it I could adjust later by reminding myself of my good fortune in getting a programme at all.

It had been left up to me to decide what level of disability I was going to demonstrate. I wanted to show the rock-bottom condition into which the illness pushed me, where I became completely rigid, unable to move my hand let alone stand up. I could just about blink, although in the end even that was replaced by a blank stare. To get into that state, however, I would have to run myself down by not taking L-dopa for four or five days. Storage would then have been completely depleted. Jan and I were on holiday in Florence until the week before filming and we had agreed that I would make an effort to be in a good state. The main problem, though, was that after filming me in the rock-bottom state on Friday, it might need more than the weekend to build up storage to demonstrate my strategies for coping. Reluctantly, I decided to give up the idea of filming the total Parkinson deficit.

So long as it didn't become too costly – by, for example, making it necessary to keep the film crew standing about idle for long periods – Patrick let me decide how I was going to manage the drug-taking. I felt that the best thing was to stay off drugs each day until the end of filming late in the afternoon and then to take quite a high dose to lay down storage for the next day.

Early on Friday morning the film crew began to arrive. A timetable had been worked out; the main constraints were the need to book the swimming pool and the university gymnasium, the availability of Jonathan (he was due to manage the Fringe at the Edinburgh Festival) and, finally, the weather. It struck me that six days was an extraordinarily tight schedule with little room for things to go wrong.

The electrician set up a series of powerful lights in the sitting room. Jonathan was expected at eleven for the first session, which would be him interviewing me. I asked Patrick if there were likely to be difficulties in recording my voice. He shrugged it off, saying that I shouldn't bother myself with any of the technicalities. But, since I'd asked, they could use sub-titles if necessary!

In spite of Patrick's reassurances that there was no need whatsoever to tidy the house for the sake of the film, as it wouldn't show up anyway, Jan had spent some time clearing things away and moving the odd bit of furniture. Everything was ready well before Jonathan was due to arrive and Patrick again raised with Jan the question of her participation. She had strong feelings about television intruding on people's private lives; she was wary of anything that even hinted at voyeurism and chose not to take part at all. I didn't mind – perhaps I preferred it that way. The programme was going to concentrate on my ideas and my explorations for an understanding of the illness, rather than be a story about my daily life in a family setting.

It was a pity things were starting so late in the day when the main benefit from storage would have been used up. Patrick promised that in spite of the expense he would get everybody to stay in Cambridge overnight so that we could do the early-morning running sequence at half-past six. Chris Morphet, the cameraman, tried out a number of positions while I sat centre stage in my cushioned armchair, loving every minute now that things were happening at last.

Within three minutes of Jonathan's arrival filming was underway. He showed the same genuine fascination with my movements and my explanations for them as he had done before. We discussed how and why I came to have this bizarre condition, what it felt like, how it affected my relations with other people and particularly the way in which I dealt with their embarrassment. I enjoyed the natural atmosphere in which the film was being made. We sat there for over an hour with no interference from Patrick and no breakdowns of equipment, which might have upset me and possibly ruined the high pitch of concentration that was demanded for a conversation with Jonathan.

At one point he could no longer resist commenting that throughout our conversation my left hand had been pummeling my lap. 'Is there any risk of your injuring yourself when you do that?' he asked.

I explained that I had sufficient control not to hurt myself, although I ran the risk of inducing an erection, which could be embarrassing.

I was completely immersed in the spirit of the occasion. There was a camera a couple of feet away and a hand-held microphone just above my head. The lights caused me to sweat gently but I ignored everything and concentrated on getting over as much as possible.

Everybody was pleased with the way the first morning had gone. On Monday, while Jonathan was in Edinburgh, filming continued, this time recording me taking a shower and getting dressed. I was very impressed by the producer's concern for naturalness and we rarely did more than one 'take'.

The crew did a brilliant job of converting day to night to give the impression that it was five o'clock in the morning, with me supposedly asleep. I succeeded in getting calm, but could feel the fingers of my left hand twitching slightly. I was concerned that this would give the impression that the tremor continued while I slept. I'd never checked, but I was pretty sure that the tremor did stop during sleep.

The shower scene was particularly good in showing my ability to redistribute the tremor: under control to squeeze shampoo on to my hair, and going berserk to whip up the shampoo into a fine lather. I used the same technique for cleaning my teeth. During filming this I pushed myself to the limits and nearly banged a couple of teeth out!

The weather was perfect for shooting the running sequence a few days later. The air by the river was cold, but the light could not have been better as the sun flooded the meadows and helped keep me dry. They used a single hand-held camera. I was left to run in whatever direction I wanted. I made off into the distance without knowing whether I was being filmed or not.

A policeman arrived. Apparently there is some rule about informing the local police station when any filming is being done outdoors. The crew tried to persuade him to walk over to speak to me but, either through shyness or because it might get him into trouble with his superiors, he refused.

I ran into a herd of cows and, still not knowing whether they were filming or not, picked some straw off the ground and proffered my shaking hand. They stared at me as they backed away. I thought it would be a good romantic touch. When I watched the rushes later, instead of feeding the cows it looked as if I was wiping their rumps!

Steam was beginning to rise from my T-shirt. We changed location. Jonathan sauntered up; immediately he grasped the atmosphere and was able to turn to advantage the opportunities that the situation offered. With no preparation or rehearsal, he judged correctly exactly what issues to raise and, as he swayed and twisted his gesturing arms this way and that, we filmed my falling forwards, jumping and running backwards, reaching up for branches from the bushes, falling against a wall and getting stuck in the process.

Jonathan had read somewhere about an experiment on a dog conducted a couple of hundred years ago. Brain damage had caused complete lack of muscle control in the animal. The experimenter threw it into a large tub of water and was amazed that the dog swam fluently. When it was back on dry land, however, it immediately returned to its previous state of immobility. Jonathan had had the bright idea that I might play the role of the dog.

Patrick had enquired about using the local swimming pool and, by coincidence, on the day that we wanted it the pool was closed to the public following its annual cleaning, so we could have it to ourselves. At eleven o'clock on Friday we duly arrived. Mimi, Patrick's assistant, changed me into my swimming costume and I kept warm by running round the edge of the pool. There were two cameras, one positioned on the high diving board and the other for use underwater.

At a nod from Patrick I positioned myself at the edge of the deep end, my back curved over, hands behind my back ready to spring into the void. With no justification, I felt completely confident that I was going to be able to swim; I thought Patrick had unnecessarily arranged for a life-saver to be on hand in case of emergencies. I started breathing in deeply and practised strokes with my arms. I felt as if all my joints were loose and rattling and my legs had gone stiff.

If I didn't go now I never would. I took a huge breath, my legs taking the strain of this unfamiliar use of my lungs. I slowly tilted forwards and, as if from nowhere, more energy pumped into my legs and ankles. Springing and falling I left the side, stretched out in the air and smacked into the water with a racing dive rather than a belly-flop.

All further thought gave way to an ecstatic feeling of fluency as my arms and legs moved in rhythmic harmony in a powerful crawl, speeding me along through the water. In no time I had reached the other side of the pool and was holding on to the side. I wanted to tell everybody about the experience and called out to Jonathan, 'It's fantastic. I swam perfectly and can you hear my voice, how loud it is? I'm coming back across.'

With ease I held on to the bar with my left hand and then positioned my feet against the tiles. I knew I would reach the other side easily. Making full use of my new-found energy, I pushed off forcefully and kept up a powerful stroke until my hand touched the bar opposite.

After moving along to the steps, I tried to get out of the pool and discovered I could hardly lift one leg above the other. My arms were virtually useless for pulling myself up. I stood suspended, with the water up to my waist and my feet gripping the steps let into the tiles. Very slowly at first, I alternately straightened up and sat back in the water until I built up momentum. When I reached a speed that I thought would work, I jettisoned myself to the top of the steps. Slowly I bent forwards, frozen with my hands locked round the rails. Jonathan was quick to see the visual impact that an interview with me in this position could provide and bent over me, like an archaeologist examining a sculpture freshly dredged from the sea.

Jonathan dried me down and I found I could move again. Surely this rigidity was linked to body temperature? If I could get the temperature of the water just right, perhaps I could carry on swimming for ages. I broke into a run and headed for the shower. The water was extremely hot, but just bearable. After a few minutes I walked out, ready for more filming. I repeated the previous dive and played around with different strokes, even attempting the butterfly, which I was able to do better than ever before. I became so confident that I did a series of dives off the springboard. Chris was kept busy, darting about underwater in his wet-suit and flippers to capture the fluent movement I was displaying.

I had been in and out of the shower a couple of times and was feeling exhausted from the repeated alternation of extreme temperatures. Patrick asked if I would like to swim across once more. This time I felt different: my movements were sluggish, my body seemed heavier. As my arms came round out of the water, my hands began to flap before calming down again on re-entry. I changed to side-stroke because I was finding it difficult to stretch my neck muscles to keep my head above the water. I reached the other side and began to have doubts about whether I should set off again. I dismissed them and slowly edged myself away from the side.

It was difficult to maintain an extended posture or to move my legs, which were beginning to sink beneath my body. I heard Jonathan call: 'Are you all right?' I did not dare interrupt the weak pattern of movement I was struggling to keep up. Again he called out: 'Are you all right?' Perhaps I could have made it, but the anxiety in his voice affected me.

There was a splash somewhere in front of me. The ripples of water spread out and struck my face. I began to swallow water. A calm voice within me declared, 'I'm going under!' The next moment a pair of hands was pushing me up to the surface. Now they were clasping my head. I realised that I was being life-saved. Secure in that knowledge, all thoughts of danger and risk to my life vanished and I called out: 'Did you get that on film?'

I was helped towards the steps, pulled up and placed in a chair.

'Maybe what's happening is that the water provides a bonus of muscular support which boosts my fluency to start with, but this is eventually lost through a drain on resources because the cold . . .'

The next day's filming was in the gymnasium. I got the impression that the BBC had only to wave its magic wand and any request for facilities would be granted immediately. By the time I arrived, Jonathan and Patrick had already selected a few pieces of equipment for me to use. We started by throwing a tennis ball to each other, then a balloon and finally a huge medicine-ball.

It was becoming clear what a crucial role posture played. If I had to make large adjustments or initiate changes of direction, I would lose postural control and find myself belting down the gymnasium, unable to stop until I crashed into the wall-bars.

Jonathan and I ran together, throwing the medicine-ball to each other as we went. If he threw the ball in front of me I could catch it, but in reaching out I fell into a faster and faster run and was soon dashing forwards to the inevitable crash. To catch the ball behind me I had somehow to twist my body round while running, catch the ball and continue through, using the ball's momentum to jive me round. The kinetic energy generated helped me jettison the ball back to Jonathan; control wasn't lost and I was able to keep running steadily without falling forwards.

Weightlifting was my idea. I thought it would provide an excellent example of what I was able to do on and off the drugs. The bar was quite heavy. On the first try off the drugs I got it as far as my knees. I tried again. Instead of signalling: 'He's trying something difficult; rustle up some resources to help,' my brain screamed: 'Stop this fool from going ahead and tearing himself apart!' I couldn't move the bar at all. Later, after the drugs had worked, I tried again and raised it as far as my head. I rested, then attempted a snatch, but the chemical was too labile and I failed to get the bar above my head. I was deeply disappointed.

*

The final piece of filming was a conversation between Jonathan and me about my attitude to L-dopa. I was very concerned to avoid giving the impression that I felt the drugs were a waste of time. I don't like having to take them, but recognise that they are a brilliant discovery and that, although I might prefer to rely on storage, without the drugs there would be no storage to draw on.

The filming concluded, the whole crew, Jan and I celebrated at a local restaurant. It wasn't long before Jonathan was regaling us with hilarious tales, filling out his descriptions richly with mime and gesture. His imitations of different actors playing Shakespeare were priceless.

We had been warned that the last thing you should do is let a film crew loose in your house. But they were a terrific lot and I don't think it was just luck that everything went so well.

The Edited Film

Within a couple of days all traces of filming had disappeared and life was back to normal. I sat in my chair, got out my checklist and tried to decide how much of what I had wanted to convey had been filmed.

Redistribution of tremor and the trade-off between tremor, rigidity and slowness of movement had been covered. Tactics for achieving temporary fluency were well illustrated. My 'mechanical bounce' came over clearly when I dropped my hand to the ground while holding a milk bottle to summon enough control to put it into the fridge. There were many instances of deceiving myself into treating acts as unimportant, and examples of interruption to smooth ballistic action.

Some detailed points hadn't been covered. I wished we'd shown how the effort to speak can cause elision, so that 'I must send a telegram' becomes 'I must send a tram'. Jonathan had seemed interested in my ideas on memory, but I should have clarified my model of arousal, emotion and motivation. All in all, I felt there was quite a lot we hadn't covered.

I wondered how long a programme Patrick would persuade the BBC to take. It had finally dawned on me that if we had done eleven hours' filming, an awful lot was going to be left out.

While we had been filming, Jonathan had suggested 'Festina Lente' as a title for the programme, but the general feeling had been that this was too obscure. Now it became apparent in a letter from Patrick that he had decided to call it simply 'Ivan'.

Patrick had been a bit vague when I had sought reassurance that I would be able to take part in the editing. Perhaps it was a good idea to have an editor who was completely separate from the producer and actors, who would probably find it impossible to be sufficiently ruthless in cutting. However, I insisted on at least seeing the rough version so that if any major points had been omitted or any distortions included, I might have a chance to persuade them to make alterations.

I received a letter from Patrick telling me that the editing was going well; I immediately rang him and asked if I could come to see how they were doing. He was very reluctant but agreed all the same.

His office and studio were high up in a converted warehouse in Chelsea, overlooking the Thames. It was enjoyable meeting again and I was introduced to the editor, Krystina. She seemed very concerned about my opinion of what she'd done. I was left alone; the familiar *Horizon* theme tune faded out and there I was in full colour running across the meadows. I was excited and apprehensive.

'That's a good bit where I'm swinging on those bars on the bridge across the stream. The colour is smashing.'

They'd kept the sequence showing me running along the edge of the field alongside Grantchester Road. I didn't usually bend forwards quite as much as that; my feet had been weighed down by clods of soil clinging to my shoes and eventually I had fallen on to my hands, which had happened only once before.

The six or seven scenes passed before my eyes. I thought the porridge-eating sequence went on too long. On the other hand, it was a good idea to try to convey to the viewer a sense of the tedium and frustration that people with Parkinson's sometimes have to endure.

'Wait a minute, though! What's this film supposed to be doing?'

I realised that I was being seduced by a brilliant piece of editing into accepting the story-angle that focused on how a person with Parkinson's disease coped, whereas I was much more interested in getting across my attempts to understand the nature of the illness for which the various scenes were supposed to provide illustrations. Soon I was spotting what had been omitted.

'Virtually the whole of the first day's filming is missing. That was when Jonathan and I covered the main theoretical points!'

The whole gymnasium scene had been dropped, apart from a brief bit of discussion at the end. The time between swimming fluently and half drowning was far too short and I felt that the impression it gave would lead people to dismiss my idea about the cold slowly creeping over me and undermining my control.

I ended up with totally mixed feelings. As a portrayal of myself with Parkinson's I thought it was entertaining, lovely to look at and very well edited; but as a scientific document it had a couple of avoidable flaws. Suddenly I realised that Jonathan's commentary was still to be superimposed. That made me feel better, because it could be used to right the balance and correct any wrong impressions.

Krystina came into the room and as she walked towards me I decided not to burden her with my points of criticism.

'You've done a marvellous job,' I said, and described in detail what I found so good about it. She stood there embarrassed but very happy.

Dialogue with Jonathan Miller

'Ivan, you've done a sort of pharmacological striptease?'

'Well, yes, but it's not rock bottom yet.'

'When was the last time you took any drugs?'

'About fourteen hours ago.'

'About how long does it take to get to base level?'

'The real rock bottom is when I stop taking medication for ten days. Then I'm lying flat out in a pool of sweat and I can't raise my little finger.'

'So this is the halfway house?'

'Exactly.'

'Let's try and break down the disability. Shaking or tremor is obviously the thing *we* notice most – but subjectively what do *you* notice?'

'For certain tasks, like speaking to you, I have to control the tremor, because it will prevent me from speaking. But in trying to control it, rigidity sets in.'

'So there's some sort of reciprocal relationship between the amount of shaking and the amount of rigidity?'

'Exactly. I can stop the shaking in two ways. One is to relax and the other is to trade off tremor for rigidity.'

'So relaxation allows you to escape the trap of having to trade off tremor and rigidity?'

'Yes, sometimes, in some circumstances. I use the ploy of holding the tremor, which if continued would induce rigidity. Then I quickly switch to a relaxing mode which is designed to reduce the basis of the tremor. It's a chicken-and-egg problem. To lose the tremor without rigidity I need to relax, but to relax I have to lose the tremor. So I hold it just long enough to intervene.'

'Do you have to use some sort of psychological trick as well to drive in the wedge of relaxation?'

'Yes. The trick is to repeat nonsense to myself.'

'A sort of secular mantra?'

'That's right.'

'What is it that you feel yourself doing when you break into the tremor?'

'I have to get rid of the tremor by smacking it out of the affected arm and by changing the pace. In other words, I try and change the speed and amplitude of the tremor from quick, short shakes to longer, slower movements which are easier to break into. This spreads the tremor more thinly throughout the body. As I slow down my arm, my feet start going faster.'

'Right, you're slowing down. Bonk, bonk, bonk. Now that ritual touching to the wings of the chair – why do you do that? There is obviously no mechanical support.'

'I don't know if I need to touch exactly. I think I probably do it to mark the end of a stage, of a journey if you like. I have to break actions down into short stages. If I think about the end goal, the emotion interferes with the action. For example, if an unknown was beating the world champion in a tennis tournament and then became conscious that it was the world champion she was playing, she might begin to fumble her shots. In terms of excitement, then, I'm in the world championship of mini-goals.'

'If you grip too long rigidity sets in?'

'Yes. I've got to beat this in a race against time, between the rigidity setting in and inducing relaxation.'

'What stops you doing this all the time?'

'Doing what?'

'If driving a wedge of relaxation into the condition, even with what seems a superhuman effort, serves to control the tremor, I suppose an unkind spectator might ask: "Why don't you do it all the time?" '

'Because I can't always make it work. The fact that you can do something once is jumped on as evidence of capability. But it might be all the control you can muster.'

'That's been your big semi-final win of the day, as it were?'

'Yes. In hospital a patient might manage to eat one or two spoonfuls on his own and is left to feed himself on the assumption that if he can do it once then hunger will produce the magical will-power to enable him to finish the meal.'

'This question may be completely unanswerable. You'll remember that Wittgenstein once asked what it is that makes the difference between the two sentences: "My hand goes up" and "I lift my hand". When you interrupt the rhythm of the tremor in a particular limb, you say you choose some muscle. Now we may know the name of the muscle, but we can't direct individual muscles merely because we know their names. We just lift our hands and that's that!'

'I don't tackle it directly. I come on it subtly, as if I was creeping up on some phenomenon. It's almost like striking a bargain with the tremor. By choosing deeper, fuller strokes, the tremor slows itself down.'

'So having struck this mysterious bargain, you go through this mantra?'

'I surprise it by cheating. Often before attempting to push it into this voluntary control, I have to give the tremor a heightened go, to give it full rein, a super chance to express itself – and then it's as if it gets fatigued and I catch it out and overlay it with voluntary control.'

'So, you've tired it out and then climbed on top of it? But I've noticed there's no way you can get from your lap to the wing of the chair other than through this ritual excursion.'

'Exactly. They're further developments of tricks to accomplish the action without my central awareness. I'm obviously aware of the goal, but it's at such a ghostly level, such a faint line in the distance, that my movements towards it are subsidiary and so far removed from it that arousal doesn't take place. It's as if to achieve a goal I have to translate the achievement into incidental movements. I have to develop a special kind of passivity.'

'So those movements – those feints that you make – you've actually slowed down and you're making your way up the north face of your armchair – these feints are quite fluent and free of tremor, but they are sort of evasions of the aim.'

'If I listen to your question and start formulating an answer which seems interesting, the arousal is massively increased, as if to destroy the accomplishment of the conscious aim.'

'So what you're trying to do is to accomplish aims while deceiving yourself into thinking that you're not?'

'That's right. It also fits my personality. I seem to have spent my life trying to be subtly successful, but not too successful because I might lose sight of the personality and attributes I like.'

'That mirrors what happens when you try to succeed in controlling the tremor. You have an enormous obstacle which would involve super-human effort to achieve directly but can be accomplished by pretending you're not really committed to it.'

'Dead right! Breaking down a movement into a series of stages makes it less effortful and the accomplishment of each stage is more feasible. Yet, paradoxically, if some movement is interrupted and broken into smaller stages in mid-air, it ruins the action and is totally debilitating.'

'So there is a distinction between predictable interruptions which divide the task into a series of subsets and unpredictable interruptions which simply disrupt the rhythm altogether?'

'Yes.'

'It's repeatedly mentioned in the literature on Parkinson's disease that patients have to divide tasks and set sub-goals.'

'I agree with that, but it also depends on what happens at the "staging post". Let's say I've broken an act into three stages and get delayed between one stage and the next. Then I may have to break the next stage down into sub-stages. This can then spiral into smaller and smaller actions, until I end up giving up the goal altogether.'

'A kind of infinite regression.'

'The crucial things are whether I've got the resources for the initiating explosion required to launch the movement at all, and how powerful that launch can be. And, as we've mentioned, it can then get complicated by the emotional attachment that may be invested in the goal.

'What I have to do is translate complex acts into one-off ballistic movements. For example, when I'm getting my breakfast I can assess very accurately the stages needed to get the components of the meal to the table. What I can't assess are unexpected interruptions, like someone coming to the door, which can make me keel over and frantically have to put the milk bottle on the floor before I spill it. Getting the bottle up from the floor may then be much more difficult than getting it from the fridge.'

'What's happened now?'

'I've held on too long at the staging post and got rigidity.'

'You were dividing the journey from your lap to the wing of the chair at a staging post by touching your lip, and you stayed too long?'

'And the tremor broke out with even greater force than ever to punish me for shutting it out.'

'So the tremor gets its own back?'

'That's right!'

'So these subdivisions of the task depend on moving very lightly and quickly, rather like moving on a series of stepping stones across a stream. It's fine as long as you dance very rapidly from one to another, but if you stop you fall in the water.'

'Yes, very good.'

'You have a letter to open, which you have some sort of apprehension about?'

'Yes. It came this morning and is to do with the sale of my sister's flat in London, which I've been trying to sell for a very long time. This may mean that the prospective buyers have pulled out.'

'So you have several things to do?'

'Until I get to the letter, I've got to shut out all thoughts about it.'

'You've got to put your glasses on, haven't you?'

'If you want me to get up at all, you'll have to keep quiet.'

'OK, so I'll shut up while you get the letter.'

'I've got to put my glasses on. I'm virtually certain I can't do it. The risks I take with the glasses exacerbate the tremor and make it more difficult to avoid being clumsy. It's beneficial to stay stooped like this. It's less effort than standing upright, so resources are available. No I can't do it . . .'

'Is there anything I can do to help or is it completely out of place to suggest?'

'I'll keep trying to do it.'

'I don't know about you sweating – I'm drenched!'

'That's it! Now let's look at the dreaded letter.'

'You mean while you were putting your glasses on you weren't thinking about the letter?'

'I couldn't possibly have thought about the letter and put my glasses on at the same time.'

'You were able to lift the letter from the mantelpiece with complete fluency. How?'

'I played a trick on myself. I pretended I was going to look at the way it was sealed.'

'In the middle of that awful shenanigans with the glasses, which was almost as painful for me as it was for you, you chucked the glasses on to your chair with accuracy and finesse and great fluency. There was no tremor at all. Someone watching might say, "Well if he can do that, why couldn't he just simply put the glasses on?" So what is it that enables you suddenly to throw the glasses?'

'It's a shift out of the arousal context.'

'A kind of playful interlude in the middle of something serious?'

'Yes. It doesn't figure, though. It was definitely part of the overall behaviour, just as getting out of the chair was.'

'Fluency seems to come back when you undertake a rather explosive movement – when you do something that involves some sort of momentum at the beginning. You seem to hitch-hike on events by jumping on movements or initiatives which lie outside your own control.'

'I prefer a more mechanical explanation. Immediately prior to throwing the glasses I was very tense and highly emotionally charged towards the goal.'

'What goal! Opening the letter?'

'No, putting the glasses on.'

'Just putting the glasses on!'

'The act of throwing the glasses wasn't so much light relief as a change to a larger, more sweeping act from the finer movements which required concentration. The release from concentration may have afforded a release of resources for smooth performance of the larger act. Concentration involves focusing, paying attention and holding at bay everything that could interfere.'

'Does music help at all?'

'If I'm stuck with, say, intense tremor, long sweeping waves of music, slow predictable music, helps induce calm and also provides, as you so beautifully put it, a pattern of sound on to which I might hitch a lift and thereby induce a slowing of the tremor to a rate at which I can impose conscious control. On the other hand, if the tremor has become locked on to a particular rhythm of music, a piece of seemingly random Stockhausen may serve to break the spell.'

'This may seem an embarrassing question – it's to do with the way you talk in some of these long explanations. You seem to get into a sort of thought rut just as you fall into a movement rut. Do you feel as if you get into a sort of recycling of thought and go over and over it again and not seem to escape from it?'

'To express my ideas I have to do it in a ballistic fashion. I've got a lot I want to say and I know I'm not going to get it over unless I blurt it out in great chunks. This reduces the number of times I have to muster the resources to start up, to initiate moving or speaking after interruption. Having once climbed aboard a wave, like a surfer, I try to stay up and keep going for as long possible.

'Now that's very difficult to achieve when I'm having a conversation that depends on feedback and modifying my ideas in the light of what my companion says. Because of concern about my failure to communicate in as clear and rich a fashion as I would like, I tend to go over the same points again and again to make sure you've got the message. Then by focusing on the component elements of an argument I may lose track of the whole idea.'

'So, in other words, do you feel that the illness affects thinking as well as motor performance or does it merely affect speech?'

'I'll answer that by suggesting that thinking is more of a motor act than is normally supposed. In the same way, motor control involves a holding operation by focusing on the relevant muscles, so thinking requires concentration, or holding at bay the continually bombarding din so that one can focus one's awareness. So the same kind of mechanism is implicated in motor acts and acts of thought, particularly in acts of memory, which thinking, of course, is heavily reliant on.'

'I've never heard the relationship of action to thought put so clearly.'

'When I'm in a low state I can't recall names or ideas and can't think richly or fluently. If I feel I'm running low on the transmitter, I try to recall the names of people in my department and if I can't then I know I'm desperately close to losing muscular control. Conversely, when I've taken a lot of medication I can lecture fluently without notes, invite questions and cope with interruption.

'Other parallels can be drawn. I told you how I might start out with an idea for action. It may then be carried out automatically or, if that's not possible, become a commitment or intention with the stakes being raised accordingly. At this point the demands upon my coping may be too great and initiating the action may be impossible, or tremor might interrupt. Somehow the act has to get off the ground. I have to interrupt the interrupting tremor or step aside from the block upon getting underway. The way to achieve this is to step sideways and convert the act into something casual or trivial. Now the lovely thing is that the same sort of approach works when you are trying to recall something from memory and you know it's there but you can't muster the means to push it forwards into consciousness. It's stuck at the amber light. It's on the tip of your tongue. What can be done? Well, you step aside and approach it indirectly. You think about doing something completely different, something that is emotionally neutral or relaxing. Then suddenly you return your attention to what it is you are trying to remember. And usually it works. You may set out to imagine a context or scene in which to place the person or object. You may start going through letters of the alphabet. However, very often remembering occurs before any ploy of this kind has been taken very far.

'Last time we met you used the phrase "pedantic perseveration" to describe the way I speak. I think the pedantry can be traced back to doing Latin at school. I do have a compulsive need to qualify everything I say in an attempt to define more precisely my ideas about complex phenomena. And the obsessive rigour subverts the intention of clarity as the idea becomes lost in a morass of amendment, anomaly, correction and elaboration, like the nesting sub-clauses of a Latin exercise.

'Perhaps the best way of characterising pedantic perseveration is to regard it as a kind of "thought tremor" equivalent to muscular tremor in the way that the expression of ideas gets locked or trapped in a repetitive cycle. The elaboration, paraphrasing and preoccupation with detail result from the search for a plausible excuse to put off the effort of interrupting the tremor of ideas and initiating a new direction of thought.

'We've just talked about perseveration as a way of squeezing as much as possible out of the energy required for launching an idea. The exigency to paraphrase and repeat everything I say may be to provide a smooth bridge to other points I want to make. I seem to be trying to launch further ideas on the strength of the previous sentence.

'But above all it may be a desire to prevent the other person talking. I feel insecure about my ability to assimilate what you say and be able to resume my train of thought. I want, above all, to offload my ideas, not to have to accommodate new ones. Far from being receptive to others' ideas as my philosophy of openness dictates, I am trying to prevent you getting a word in edgeways!'

'All this is a very elaborate way of not reading the letter!'

'Now the salient thing is the content of the letter. I'm really only concerned about what it's going to say . . .'

'Is it good news?'

'It seems they do intend to proceed . . . anyway, the main thing is it's all right.'

'The way you threw the envelope – the fluency with which you threw it away – the one thing that didn't matter; and then the extraordinary tremor as you read the letter – the one thing that did matter.'

'It's as if getting rid of the envelope was hardly an act because it was not given a goal – it was literally a throwaway act – decoupled from the goal of reading the letter.'

'Cut!' said Patrick. 'That gives us more than enough.'

Going to the Cinema

Going to the cinema was one of the pleasures I was very reluctant to give up. The first hurdle was getting there. Off the drugs it was a terrible strain to walk the mile or so; it was best if I had somehow engineered a good state of storage or was prepared to be on the drugs in time for setting out. The worst thing that could happen was for the drugs not to have 'taken'. This would then mean a journey fraught with strain for Jan as well as for me, as I would have to walk with my hands clasped behind my back while Jan pushed down on my locked fingers to prevent me keeling over. There were taxis, but we liked to go to the pictures quite a lot and it was too expensive to pay for a taxi every time.

On this particular occasion I had taken a small amount of drugs in the hope of avoiding another problem, which often occurred after I took a large dose: falling asleep and missing most of the film. The small dose had worked and we were more than halfway there, chatting happily as we walked along. We entered the Market Square and saw the long queue for the film at the Victoria Cinema. Just as I was hoping we wouldn't meet anyone we knew, I suddenly lost control. Jan quickly held my hands in position and gently frog-marched me to our film at the Arts Cinema.

Jan had already cycled in to buy the tickets in advance, but a smooth passage through the cinema to our seats was interrupted by another disabled person who was struggling to get through the swing doors with his crutches. We were behind him, and he turned round and asked if I would mind holding the door open. I was standing on my own, waiting for Jan to return from the loo. I had compressed all my tremor into rigidity. I told him I was very sorry but I couldn't help him, and then made the fatal admission that I had Parkinson's disease. As soon as I heard the words, the rigidity was transformed into violent shaking.

The pair of us completely blocked the entrance, unable to disentangle ourselves from an ever-tightening knot of crutches and limbs. Jan arrived back upstairs, eased her way through the throng of people and hauled me into an upright position. We broke the deadlock of who should go first by my tumbling forwards past an officious ticket collector.

Keeping my gaze to the floor to avoid eye contact and the crippling effect of expressions of sympathy or embarrassment, I scrambled to my seat. It was at the end of a row, which enabled me to stretch my legs out into the aisle. Jan sat down beside me and asked if I was OK. I replied that I was, but the force of my tremor was making the row of seats tremble. I tried to make light of the possible disturbance I might be causing. I imagined people asking for 'emotional' seats as word got round that there were some which vibrated to allow you to experience the film's changing emotional tone.

The lights had dimmed when a woman came and stood next to me, waiting for me to get up to let her go past. I was completely frozen and couldn't begin to move. Jan hadn't yet noticed her and I turned to the woman and managed to whisper, 'I'm sorry, I can't move.'

Jan looked to see what I wanted, saw the woman and repeated that I couldn't move and would she please go round to the other aisle.

'What do you mean, he can't move! How did he get here, then?'

Jan leaned over further and whispered, 'I'm sorry, but you'll have to go round to the other end.'

After hovering there for what seemed like minutes, the woman decided to have a go at getting past. She tried to force my legs to one side by pushing against my knees, but the Parkinsonian lock was too much for her. So she tried to step over them. With a lot of grumbling she finally got past and clumsily stomped her way to the vacant seat.

It took me about ten minutes to calm down and establish reasonable control over the tremor. I tried to concentrate on the film but my mind kept wandering to another occasion when I had been paralysed at the pictures – but that time it had been with adolescent embarrassment as I went through agonies mustering the courage to kiss a girl in the back row . . . Back in Cambridge a quarter of a century later, I suddenly realised that the film was drawing to a close. I had missed a lot of the story, but I was pleased that at least I hadn't fallen asleep.

A few minutes later the drugs worked at last, and when the film ended and the lights came on I looked over to where the woman was sitting. She was staring intently at me. I got up and walked completely fluently towards the exit, trying not to laugh at her outraged expression.

Further Conversations with Jonathan

'Do you feel that you ever have to let strangers off the hook by explaining to them: "Don't mind me. I'm shaking but I know I'm shaking, so don't think you need to be embarrassed"? There's the embarrassment of a defective performance which frustrates you and lowers your self-esteem and there is something I've experienced as a stammerer, of being embarrassed on behalf of those who are embarrassed for me. Does that ever happen to you?'

'Frequently. For example, when I feel people want to intervene, but are not quite sure how, I mobilise resources to cope with what I predict is the way they are going to intervene, which makes me shake even more.'

'Because they're going to try to help – but incompetently?'

'Perhaps. It's not really embarrassment, though, so much as an exacerbation of the situation. I try to anticipate the way in which they are going to act upon their embarrassment because their interventions are going to need handling.'

'Do you ever feel that it would help, when you meet someone for the first time, for them to be given a printed manifesto of what they're about to see so that at least that can be got out of the way. Or do you prefer to deal with it intuitively as the occasion arises?'

'Yes, spontaneously. This idea of embarrassment is interesting. At Gatwick, on the way back from Italy this summer, we had to walk the gauntlet of people waiting for relatives and friends – crowds of people smiling and waving as I hobbled through, having gone into deficit prematurely. It made me walk more and more slowly until we almost ground to a halt by the time we'd got through. When we were in Italy I wasn't concerned at all. The people we met weren't going to figure in my life and we were separated by language. It was quite a joke to watch the Italians react in their own fascinating way; if you looked round, they were huddled together pointing and chatting away.'

'I'm staring into space to keep out any possible distractions in order to get out of this chair. Even my diversionary ploys won't work because I've fallen into such a bad state. I've no resources to play with. There's an interesting tendency to laugh the more helpless I become! I don't know if it's to brighten my spirits. I suspect it's originally to ward off aggression by others who witness my weakness.

'However much I break down the goal into sub-units, I can't initiate the act. I'll try and make a big lurch – by breathing. I'll tell you if I need help. Now! Done it! That was like climbing Everest.'

'The shower gives me a fillip – an extra fluency which enables me to get washed and feel good – invigorated. I can stand upright. Once I get the soap in position, the tremor just goes to work.'

'Is this the way you usually bring your runs to an end, by running into a wall?! Is it hard to stop without finding a wall to throw yourself against?'
'No. I do this to relax the strain on my arms that builds up when I'm running. If I fall against a wall and push off quickly it reduces the rigidity.'
'If you're hesitant can you jam?'
'That often happens.'
'Now you've spent too long.'
'Yes, I'm stuck.'
'Is there anything I can do?'
'No.'
'It looks terribly painful.'
'It's a hell of a strain on the ankles and legs. I've got to get off this wall. It's pretty urgent!'
'Or what?'
'Or my head bangs against the wall repeatedly.'
'Oh yes, I see.'
'Head-banging without the glue. In the end I just have to drop to my knees, which I'm going to do now. Then I'll probably get stuck on the ground.'
'Does this often happen on your morning runs?'
'I often come to this wall.'
'Really?'
'But I try and make sure I don't fall.'
'So it's the "shaking wall of Cambridge".'
'People come and weep at this wall!'
'But you seemed completely fluent during the running.'
'I'm really stuck now. I've got a fly buzzing round my head and I'm waiting for your next question.'

'All right. I'll ask the question and swat the fly. Meeting someone with whom you have to talk is a fatal interruption on these runs, then?'

'Absolute disaster! If I meet a pretty female, I've had it. If I meet a dog, say an Alsatian, and it's not on a lead, that's a killer. When I was in Italy the farmer said to go jogging wherever I liked. This bloody great Alsatian came and grabbed my leg and I just went over like this.'

'Like that!'

'Yeh, and that probably saved me.'

'I suppose it puzzled the hell out of the dog.'

'It was probably taken as total surrender. I must straighten up – not talk any more.'

'There a competition between talking and tremor. Even people who haven't got Parkinson's can have difficulty. I've noticed that colleagues who get involved in intense conversations while walking down the corridor stop to be able to cope with the conversation. They can't walk and talk at the same time.

'In a similar way I'm trading off conversation and tremor when I'm low on drugs. On the drugs, I have to trade off conversation with writhing.'

'Perhaps I'm being over optimistic, but it sounds as if your ideas flow with more spontaneity and they don't recycle quite so much now you're on the drugs as they seem to when you're in the off state.'

'It's complicated. When I'm off, I can think clearly by trading intellectual processing for tremor or rigidity. But there comes a stage of deficit where it gets very difficult to continue to do this any more.'

'Is that because you're thinking about musculature or is it some intrinsic dissolution of the thinking?'

'There is an interference stage where I'm dealing with the tremor and distractions and it's difficult to concentrate.'

'That is a subtraction effect.'

'Exactly. But it eventually shifts to a level where it's almost impossible to hold on to ideas at all and it's as if thinking – drawing ideas into consciousness or consideration – is not succeeding because of the collapse of holding everything else at bay while I concentrate.'

'On the salient topic?'

'Yes. That's the state when I'm in deficit. When I take the drugs there is a fascinating interim phase before the drugs have taken – in the sense that the chemical hasn't flooded through the system to peripheral muscular control. If I engage in intellectual activity at this point it's as if I can siphon off the drug from the muscles to intellectual processing.

'I am at my most creative and think most fluently then. The expression of these thoughts and ideas may not be too coherent, but the actual thinking is extremely fluent.

'I'm in this awful dilemma of having fabulous thoughts and creative explosions, yet I've got tremor and can't record them. It's very difficult even to press the button on the tape-recorder. And even if I do manage to record, very few people, apart from Justin, my son, seem able to hear or understand what I've said.

'Then the medication takes and often there's an increase in motor fluency in which I can speak but I've dried up on the ideas.

'It's like a wave. Once it's shifted to the motor side it goes on drawing away the benefit – and even sets up a state of deficit – in intellectual fluency.'

I pulled out some journal articles from my files.

'Why were you able to do that so easily?'

'Well, it could be a number of things. Anything that helps disguise the act and it's attachment to a goal and thereby reduce the emotional charge; or anything that reduces the fineness of what I want to do; or involves fewer changes in directing muscles.'

'Ah, so that's why it's easier to run with those big global movements than pour the honey on the porridge, with all the careful adjusting and wrist control that needs.'

'Exactly – and anything that requires a more careful, a more intense level of holding background muscles that aren't directly involved in the act is difficult.'

'What you've told me about your difficulty concentrating – it's almost like the two parts of the retina of the eye. There are the things you focus on with great concentration in the middle – with the centre of your will and consciousness of a goal – which can exacerbate the tremor. And there are actions that aren't loaded with meaning – the things you half see out of the corner of your eye as it were – that you are able to do fluently.'

'I wonder whether the tremor would disappear if I were to adopt a life of total blandness, free of all emotional charge. I haven't found anyone to do it yet, but I want to explore the possibility of inducing a deep hypnotic trance to see if control could be suggested for the post-hypnotic state.'

'Let's try to get the difference between the two states clear.'

'My ideas about concentration must seem paradoxical. When I'm off the drugs I really enjoy being able to read the newspaper right through without distraction. I can concentrate better when I'm off the drugs. But I've also said that dopamine enables me to hold back other concerns, in other words to take the strain while I concentrate on what I want to do.'

'What's the answer, then?'

'I'm not sure, but I think that I can get the extra resources for concentrating in two ways. One is by adding supply through my existing drugs. The other is to sacrifice and give up the strain of control. I've allowed that threshold to break down. Once through that threshold, it is possible to concentrate attention. But a point is reached where the flapping arms and trembling become so great that they disrupt, and the ability to concentrate collapses.'

'I see. So up to a point it's useful to be off the drug and you can use these various techniques for soaking up the tremor, but eventually the chaos is too much?'

'Yes, that's very clear. These two states off the drug are matched by two states on the drug. Medication allows me to adopt the opposite strategy of adding resources rather than sacrificing control. I've found I'm able to lecture extremely fluently or take on highly complex activities with numerous sudden changes of direction, but, again, only up to a point. The adverse effects of the drugs – the writhing movements – become so intense as to interfere in the same way as the tremor.'

'I see what you mean. But I get the impression from what you've said on other occasions that it is a different kind of concentration when you're on the drugs.'

'Yes, that's right. The concentration when I'm off – it's as if I allow information to get in, a sort of feedback, while I ignore the background chaos. I'm receptive to the information in the newspaper.

'When I'm on the drug I'm in the luxurious position of being able to make forays into the chaos of the mind – it's a much more adventurous state – and I can grasp hold of information and incorporate it in a divergent way.'

'You mean when you're off the drugs you can concentrate in a linear, analytic way. While you're on the drugs you are able to build castles in the air and, as you said before, this creative mode is at its highest after you've taken the drugs, but before they "take" and restore control to your muscles.'

'Yes, and that is the time before the writhing and other adverse effects start up.'

'Someone seeing you from the outside might still wonder, even taking into account the writhing, why you so determinedly prefer to keep off the drugs.'

'Living off storage is totally different from coping with the concurrent goading from the drugs.'

'What exactly do you mean?'

'Exogenous drugs, rather than naturally produced dopamine, bombard the brain in amounts and at a speed which prevents the brain regulating the take up of the new dopamine. There is an imperative to take up the chemical rather than what seems to happen normally where storage or production is demanded only when needed.

'Essentially it is a supply-dominated system with drugs, rather than a demand-oriented system.'

One of the film crew mumbled, 'We've got enough for six programmes here!' and we broke for lunch.

The *Listener* Article

I am not sure if Patrick Uden had a hand in it, but soon after my visit to his studio I received an invitation from the *Listener* to write an article about my Parkinson's disease. This was my chance: the readership must include doctors and research workers. The title and opening paragraphs would be important. How about 'Out of Control with Parkinson's Disease' or 'The Man Who Couldn't Stop Moving'? I ended up with a far less dramatic title: 'The Experience of Parkinson's Disease'.

I thought carefully about the best state to be in for the task and over a period of three days built up a pile of notes and summaries I had written previously. I needed muscular control to do the physical search, the carrying and the ordering of the material.

On the fourth day I came off the drugs and, relying on a high level of storage, began to write. The ideas flowed and the whole thing began to take shape. If I started with an example of the way the deficit transformed a fairly routine activity, I could then go on to make the point that the film had shown only one particular level of Parkinsonian deficit and that there were both milder and more severe stages.

Although I knew I was greatly over-simplifying the complexity of the brain's functioning, I felt that the model I proposed was acceptable. I had to force myself to hold back from making numerous qualifications. The concept of stress that underpinned much of what I wanted to say required a definition, as did the other key issues: arousal, emotion, feedback and feedforward.

I argued that the deficit in Parkinson's, and the drug that remedied the deficit, should be identified with the notion of coping. That was self-evident and hardly an explanation. The questions to ask were: 'Coping with what?' and 'How was coping achieved? Was it by holding back the source of interference or did it provide directly the means for functions to operate?'

As I had learnt early on in my researches, dopamine is among a number of chemicals in the brain which serve to facilitate or inhibit the transmission of messages along the neural pathways. When cells for vision are stimulated by input from the environment there is a process called 'surround inhibition' whereby neighbouring cells are dampened down and the stimulated cells more readily excited by the contrast. Could transmitters such as dopamine be doing two jobs at the same time: damping down unwanted activity and also facilitating required functions? Is dopamine a chemical for holding and letting go? Or does it just do the holding while a different chemical provides the release mechanism? There seemed to be a possibility of reconciling Freud's position with mine! Stress and cell exhaustion would arise for him through protracted holding, while for me it would come through excessive demand for flow.

How could I get this over to informed readers, let alone those who knew nothing about the subject? How was I to avoid discussing the fact that there were other chemical transmitters whose role was clearly established in the functions I was convinced were affected by Parkinson's disease and the chemical dopamine?

In the scientific community it seemed to be accepted as fact that dopamine deficiency was the cause of Parkinson's. However, there were grounds for believing that other transmitters, with a close chemical relationship to dopamine, might also be in short supply. I could argue that Parkinson's disease encompassed the loss of cells producing these other chemicals or that such cells might be recruited to compensate for the shortfall of dopamine.

There was very strong evidence that memory was served by a transmitter chemically far removed from dopamine. How was I to reconcile that with my compelling experience, while off the drugs, of inability to retrieve from memory names, ideas and information which become readily accessible when I raise the brain's level of dopamine by taking L-dopa? The only answer would be to adopt a far more complex model.

I'd found that Parkinson's disease affects a wide range of functions: muscle control, memory, body-temperature regulation, planning and sexual activity. The factor common to all these was 'arousal', which I would define as a particular level of alertness which produces an emotional experience whenever there is a change in the degree of uncertainty about one's circumstances.

Throughout the seven years I'd had Parkinson's, changes in the intensity of the tremor had provided a very good indication of changes in my level of arousal. Loud noises, people entering the room, the car not starting, were the obvious triggers to such alterations, yet an effect upon muscular control did not always occur.

Planning ways of accomplishing particular goals and assessing my capability to achieve them required a check against arousal to determine whether I should become committed or not. Trying to relax and achieve calm was far easier if there were few interruptions in my auditory, visual or other sensory environment.

The model I was trying to develop went as follows. Change is registered as arousal and felt as emotion. Arousal and emotion induce the release of chemical transmitters which provide the means for coping. Parkinson's disease impairs the individual's ability to be ready to meet such change because the brain can no longer produce dopamine in sufficient quantity.

It was a couple of weeks after sending in my article to the *Listener* before I heard from the editor. He had passed it on to someone in the medical field to read and it must have been acceptable because he told me that it would be published in the same week that the *Horizon* programme was shown. I felt very pleased that at last I was getting my ideas into print and might be able to have at least a short rest from trying to understand the illness. As with the television programme, though, I lost complete control of what happened to my article once it was in the hands of the editor.

I pounced on the packet of six copies of the *Listener* that were posted through the letter-box. There was a large coloured photograph of me, which I liked. My eyes darted up to the title: 'Learning the Tactics of Coping'.

Why this emphasis on coping? They must have seen the film and felt that was the main feature that came across. It was only on the third reading that I realised a couple of sentences had been deleted. One was my suggestion that the buoyancy in the swimming baths had released resources from holding posture and thus produced the extraordinary muscular fluency. I felt annoyed! The swimming sequence raised some of the most important issues. Was the fundamental problem to do with posture and gravity? (It would be an interesting experiment to join one of the Boeing flights where the plane goes into a steep dive and you become weightless for a short time to see if I regained muscular fluency temporarily.)

'Oh, that's unfortunate! They've snipped out my acknowledgement to Professor Marsden.' This was a reference to his seminal paper in which he identified the key feature in Parkinson's disease as 'the breakdown of the automatic execution of learned motor plans'. I argued that this model might apply at one stage of the disease's progress, but at different stages other features might be more important, such as inability to initiate movement, failure to incorporate deviations into ongoing actions, deterioration of memory retrieval, or changes in ways of thinking.

I was worried that the article might give the impression that I believed there was generally a finite amount of resource which was shared out among the various functions. I thought that the picture was more complicated than that. I had not given sufficient prominence to the role of storage, which afforded a high degree of independent functioning before stress and strain revealed the ultimately finite nature of the resources. Storage was laid down in anticipation of an expected level of demand. Willingness to release resources from storage would depend upon the abundance of supply and the degree of urgency of the demand. But I was fussing over detail, and decided I must allow myself to be satisfied with the way things had gone.

Response to the Film

The reviews of the *Horizon* programme that appeared in the newspapers were excellent, but again focused too much on coping instead of on my search for understanding. I liked the piece by Benny Green in *Punch*: 'Vaughan sees himself as a kind of empirical scientist approaching the problem of his own affliction as a metaphysical puzzle to be solved or at least understood'.

In spite of my reservations about the reviews in general, though, my emotions capitulated in the face of the universally favourable response, and because I understood what Patrick and Jonathan had been trying to achieve.

I wondered what response I would have from the medical profession and the general public, and I was particularly pleased to receive a letter, within two days of the programme being shown, from Veronica Nanton, a research fellow at Birmingham University who was engaged in research into Parkinson's disease. She wrote, 'I found the programme one of the most honest accounts of the experience of Parkinson's disease that I have come across. I am sure it will have given encouragement to thousands of sufferers and their families.'

With one notable exception, there was little response from the medical profession. Iain Wilkinson wrote to congratulate me on the programme; better still, he popped round with a couple of bottles of wine. I don't think I really expected to hear from Professor Marsden's research group, who had not been brought in at any stage of the programme's development. My relationship with them was ambiguous: on the one hand I was merely a subject in their research; on the other I was determinedly carving out my own piece of territory, since this was the only way I could hope to make inroads on the traditional doctor–patient relationship. In this I had taken the path of the prodigal son and hoped that I would be welcomed back at any time. I was confident that Professor Marsden was above any professional pique. I smiled as I realised that, anyway, he had not tried to fit me into a television programme of his which had been transmitted two weeks before my *Horizon* film . . . It was a case of two entirely different approaches with very little possibility of overlap.

The Christmas issue of the Parkinson's Disease Society newsletter had already been printed before the programme went out, so when the spring issue arrived I was curious to see what it would say. When I found that there was a five-page report, my calm curiosity turned into tremulous excitement.

– Blinkin' heck! They report an estimate that thirty million people watched it. That can't be right! It's sad that they seem to have had so many phone calls and letters from people who have been upset. I wonder how many rang in to say they'd enjoyed it?

– 'Idiosyncratic approach' – that's certainly true. They talk about living 'nearly as full a life as before with modern treatment, physiotherapy and tender loving care'. I expect to carry on living a completely full life, while accepting that some adjustments have to be made. I can understand their resentment at not being contacted for guidance, though.

– This point about being 'determined to make life difficult for myself' is hardly fair. The example of the T-shirt that he refers to is an authentic illustration of the problems I face given my style of managing the drugs. He would do better to argue against that. I could use velcro like he suggests. The velcro fasteners on my running shoes are great, but aligning a velcro fastener on a coat or shirt would be very tricky.

– He says I seem 'to have isolated myself from the neurological help available'. That certainly isn't true. I see Iain regularly and we share information. I follow some of his suggestions, others I don't, and he readily accepts my active role in the management of the drugs, not only out of respect for my personality, but also through a realistic assessment that there is still a great deal of room for trial and error in establishing the best drug regime to follow.

– There's no meat in the comments from the press they quote. This criticism about 'media sensationalism' is countered rather well by the *Horizon* editor's letter they reproduce. He points out that there were two *Horizon* programmes only a couple of weeks apart, the first with the world's leading experts like Professor Marsden stressing the success of L-dopa. Our programme aimed to show my personal approach to understanding what was going on and to demonstrate that the drugs are not the magic cure.

– I feel very strongly about the moral implications of giving the general public the impression that all is now well in the treatment of Parkinson's. It makes life very difficult for sufferers of the disease when any problems that arise are attributed either to an unreasonable resistance against the drugs or else to unintentional mismanagement.

– This last point is quite nice, though: 'One thing is certain: many more thousands of people are now aware of Parkinson's disease than before . . .'.

The idea of setting up independent funding for my own research became a possibility through the publicity from the programme. I wrote to a couple of newspapers and paid them to insert the simple request: 'Support Ivan Vaughan's Parkinson's Disease Research', together with my address and telephone number. I wanted the luxury of being able to devote time and money to research projects, including those which might be regarded as unorthodox.

The BBC were very upset by so blatant an attempt to gain financially from one of their programmes. But I hadn't received any payment for doing the programme, on the ground that I had engaged the services of the BBC rather than the other way round. It had never occurred to me to ask Patrick, in the middle of filming, to tell the BBC I would be unable to carry on unless they paid me.

In the event, a total of around five hundred pounds was donated, mostly in amounts of five or ten pounds, and a charity based in the West Country generously offered four payments of two hundred and fifty pounds spread over two years.

I quickly drew up an outline of the kind of research I intended to conduct. I was particularly keen to 'search for drug strategies and conditions which succeed in laying down storage in the most efficient manner'. Overall I was interested in improving the theoretical understanding of what the illness entailed and in searching for practical ways of coping with the symptoms.

I proposed adopting my proven method of observing the effects on my behaviour of varying the management of the drugs and the environment, followed by careful analysis and introspection. In this way observation about areas of behaviour could be linked to theoretical speculation. I had managed to reduce my original list of over a hundred themes or behavioural areas but, even so, there were seventeen themes and nineteen theoretical constructs.

One of the many people who wrote to me was John Williams, a lecturer in pharmacology at Bristol University. He'd had Parkinson's disease for six years and was also keen to do some research. I invited him to stay for the weekend and was very impressed by his condition, especially the constancy of his state throughout the day. Until a few months before he had been on the same combination of L-dopa and Carbidopa as myself.

Then he had started taking a new drug called Eldepryl which he highly recommended.

However, I wasn't ready to change my drugs. What did this drug think it was doing, coming along and disturbing my equilibrium! I decided to check the literature to find out the risks and adverse reactions which were bound to exist, and it was only apparent in retrospect how I magnified the adverse effects of the new drug and played down its benefits. Perhaps I was adopting Karl Popper's sound scientific principle of seeking to refute a hypothesis, but I knew I was deceiving myself. The hypothesis I wanted to undermine was someone else's and I was attacking it in order to confirm and sustain my own approach.

John paid us a second visit later in the year and brought along a large number of containers for collecting urine samples. He wanted me to fill one a day for a week, parcel them up and post them back to him for analysis. Jan had to take samples as well to act as a control subject. The most memorable event of his stay was Sophie's cry of disgust at finding the salad compartment of the fridge full of row upon row of sample bottles containing the patently obvious orange liquid!

I was kept fully occupied at college during the spring and summer terms. During the Easter vacation, however, I attended a conference on Parkinson's disease organised by the Eastern Motor Group. I was invited to speak under the broad heading of 'My Experience of Parkinson's'. I was given forty minutes at the beginning of the afternoon session at two o'clock.

To be in my best state for delivering the talk, I held off the medication until lunchtime, as writhing was usually absent during the period of the first dose of drugs. I was interested in the morning sessions and arrived by taxi at ten o'clock. I was able to walk but couldn't stand up for very long, particularly if someone came over and talked to me. I was shaking quite a lot and in order not to distract the speaker I ostracised myself to one of the corners at the back of the lecture theatre.

Towards the end of the morning I was in quite a bad way. I couldn't possibly join the others for lunch and, although I'd anticipated this happening and had brought along some honey sandwiches, I couldn't help a twinge of sadness at being stuck in a chair on my own for an hour and a half, using all my skill to ensure that the drugs were timed exactly right. If they worked too soon the benefit would be wasted, too late and I would be in a real mess.

At a quarter to two the conference organiser came to see how I was and very wisely reassured me that it didn't matter in the least if I wasn't ready by two o'clock. They could easily ask the speaker who was due after me to go first. That calmed me down considerably, although the sight of people returning to their seats reminded me forcibly of the fast approaching deadline.

At a couple of minutes past two I felt the sluice gates open, at least enough to give me confidence to walk down to the platform, sit in a chair and let the audience know that I had not stage-managed my predicament. For those who had not seen it before, the transition from the 'off' to the 'on' state should be interesting. I squeezed my fingers together, contorted my body into different positions and relaxed with my hands on my knees. A second later I stood up, stretched and began an account of how my day might be spent from waking at five o'clock to bedtime at ten thirty. I explained that to give my talk I'd taken quite a high dose of drugs but that if I'd taken them earlier I would almost certainly have had to battle to prevent myself being distracted by severe writhing movements, generally known as dyskinesias.

I described how difficult it was to keep my thoughts in check while I spoke – not in the sense of holding back irrelevancies, but rather of preventing my mind from racing ahead of my delivery to construct new ideas related to the theme in hand, but off at creative tangents.

'In his talk this morning Ken Flowers described his experiments on "mental set". Now, there is one thing that needs clarification – and as I say that I realise that the drugs have given me sufficient confidence to start without any idea of what this point about Ken's work is going to be! As I talk about the process whereby my thoughts are converted into utterances, my brain is busy shunting forwards the words and the grammar for making the ideas intelligible and simultaneously reviewing Ken's talk for the points I want to make. Instead of waiting until I have securely formulated what I want to say, I am able to take risks and leap out into space, drawing along the supporting bridge as I go. Mind you, there are limits to this, and I'm not sure if I'm going to be able to remember what my point of criticism was! I've gone too far and am stalling for time.

'Ah! Here it comes – that's it! Ken fails to consider that the subjects in his experiments were all on medication. The drugs are taken to restore function. My experience is that, when taken in the recommended dosage, as is the case of Ken's subjects, the drugs come very close to eliminating the deficit of Parkinson's. So any difference in the scores between the normal group and the Parkinson patients may be owing to adverse reactions from the drugs.

'I find that the drugs can produce a better state than normal for performing all sorts of tasks, providing that control isn't undermined by the quite different adverse reactions from the drugs. What is needed is a study of individual differences related to the response to the medication and the nature of the task.'

A month later I received a letter from Dr David Lee, a psychologist at Edinburgh University. He invited me to go and stay for three or four days. There was no formal programme of events, but we thought we might try a bit of filming. I managed the train journey to Edinburgh successfully and was met by Martin Frischer, one of David Lee's research students, who was going to put me up in his flat and generally look after me. I very much enjoyed being back in Edinburgh, which I had visited once before. I was able to go for early morning runs and would stay off my drugs for most of the day, trying to sustain the level of background storage by taking quite a lot in the late afternoon and evening.

The television studio was available throughout my stay and we covered a lot of the same ground as in the *Horizon* film. One new feature, however, was trampolining. The day we filmed that, I had been off my drugs all day. At three o'clock I launched myself on to a huge trampoline, which had been set up specially in a large hall. After a lot of bouncing, falling and springing, I eventually came off and then spent an exciting hour playing football, excitedly rushing round, darting in different directions, all with perfect postural control.

It was as puzzling as the fluency when I went swimming for the *Horizon* programme. Perhaps the trampolining had induced my brain to release resources usually retained for the very extremes of shock. I didn't know what to make of it. Equally puzzling was the way I ran two days later back in Cambridge.

The morning after my return from Edinburgh I set out as usual for my run. There is a triangular field near home measuring approximately half a mile round. I felt confident and the weather was good: soon the sun would be warming the far side of the track and would help dry me out. I skipped across the A10. I wasn't at all bothered by the three horses that had walked through from Coe Fen and I completed two laps without any muscular or psychological tension. I didn't have any particular goal in mind, but was just enjoying the physical activity. I kept going and did another three laps.

The horses reminded me of a visit to Meldreth School for children with cerebral palsy, a few miles south of Cambridge, where there are excellent facilities for swimming and also for riding, which was what I was going to do there. I was off my drugs but the horse was completely docile; it wasn't in the least disturbed as I mawled it's neck, repeatedly stabbed it with my feet and gave it a most unpredictable and confusing set of signals. I was interested to see if I could latch on to the horse's rhythm and release part of the resources committed to posture. However, I found that it took all my energy just to stay in the saddle. I was already giggling a bit. We had just turned a corner when my foot belted the horse particularly hard and it broke wind hugely. I burst out laughing and started to slide off . . .

I made it a rule never to cheat as I ran round the triangle and always kept to the outside of imaginary posts. I felt no pressure to cut the corners and was beginning to sense a change in the way I ran. Earlier I had been stopping and starting as usual, alternating brisk walks with the running. Now I felt I could keep going without stopping or changing my pace. My breathing was better. A cool contentment accompanied the harmony between my co-operating muscles, the match between my body temperature and the air around me. Slowly I drifted into reflection about what was happening.

– Surely this is the fully fledged aerobic rhythm that I have been trying so hard to attain. [I lost count of the number of times I had gone round.] I'm not sweating and I don't feel particularly hot. Perhaps Parkinson's is the breakdown of the anaerobic resources for initiating or changing the direction of activity.

I moved sideways in my thinking about oxygen.

– Maybe that Oxford academic, Russell, was right in his book on the brain when he warned of the danger of falling asleep while sitting upright in a chair. I'm always doing that and, combined with a reduction in the heart's functioning owing to the drugs, perhaps I was starving my brain of oxygen for all those years. Does the distinction between aerobic and anaerobic link up with the improved feeling of control I get when I drink champagne? That's the answer – raise the brain level of carbon dioxide with loads of champagne!

The traffic was building up on the A10; it didn't bother me at all. Cyclists were coming up behind me, people were walking towards me but there was no panic and no worry about holding myself together in the face of these new arrivals on my scene. Without the usual urgency and over-excitement, I switched calmly back into reverie.

As a child, instead of simply swimming, diving and jumping when I went to the local baths, I would spend considerable time trying to improve on my previous best distance swimming underwater. I had managed to hold my breath and swim up to one and three-quarter lengths. Then there was weightlifting. My approach had been to heave the weights all over the place without any concern for breathing properly.

– Energy from anaerobic sources is supposed to be drawn upon in brief spurts, each lasting no more than a couple of seconds. Have I been misusing it? Is it supposed to be reserved to supplement oxygen-based energy to deal with surprise or interruption in either activity or thought? Anaerobic resources provide the means for holding out while changes are made or felt. Have I pushed myself into situations of stress where I've chosen or been forced to hold out way beyond normal limits?

The pleasure I was feeling as I turned the corner for at least the twelfth time was different from my usual manic inclination to whoop with ecstasy. It was a much calmer flow in which energy seemed to be conserved rather than used up liberally in celebration. Round once more, then I decided to head for home.

Breakfast with Birgit

Clunk. The door burst open and Birgit swept in with her customary, 'Hello, how are you today?'

She shut the kitchen door behind her and, when I failed to respond, curbed her natural exuberance and pulled on my running shoes for me before I managed to say, 'I'm fine, not bad.'

I sat passively as this attractive, plump, fifty-two-year-old Swedish blonde completed the routine of dressing me. Occasionally she came running with me and we would skip and dance across the fens like a Laurel and Hardy double act; but not this time. I told her I was going on the medium run and that I would be back in twenty minutes.

It was six-thirty in the morning and still dark as I headed off down to the river. I enjoyed the run and arrived back twenty-five minutes later. Once inside, the change in temperature made me break into a sweat. In no time at all Birgit whipped off my track suit, T-shirt, shoes and socks. The shower was set running and I was enjoying the reduction in tension provided by the warm water. For the umpteenth time I reflected on how incredible it was for the council to have provided a grant for this walk-in shower. Soon Birgit joined me, having changed into a lightweight waterproof smock. Her hands deftly rubbed shampoo into my hair while I held on to the bars.

'You're in quite a good state today! You're able to stand more upright.'

She'd learnt not to expect much response from me while the shower was running. The chances were that anything I said would be inaudible or so delayed and abbreviated as to have lost all meaning. She rubbed the soap over my body, vigorously, efficiently and discreetly. As she went to put the shower-head back in its holder I felt soapiness under my left arm which she'd forgotten to rinse.

'You've . . . my . . .,' my lips started popping as if determined to prevent me completing what I wanted to say.

'What?'

Birgit guessed I wanted the fan-heater on. By now I was trembling with frustration. She noticed my excitement and turned to the light-switch. I looked away in an attempt to gain a moment's calm so that I could blurt out the message I wanted. Birgit interpreted the relaxation of my gaze as a signal to go ahead and pulled the light-cord.

'My arm . . . soapy!' I puffed out.

But it was too late. The light came on and the automatic fan extracted the warm air and drew in cold from under the door.

'Which arm?'

I turned my head and stared at my left shoulder. I brought round my right hand and stabbed the spot.

'Please shower the soap away from here,' I said easily. Hoping to take advantage of the momentary restoration of fluency, I piled on the instructions. 'Can you put the heater on? Could we try drying my hair first this time? I'm afraid there's no mushrooms!'

I was eager to get past the emotion associated with disappointing news. Birgit got tremendous pleasure from feeding me as large and varied a breakfast as possible.

'You've got bacon and tomatoes though, haven't you? There should be eggs. There were over a dozen last time I came.'

'Yes, there were.'

I was soon dry through the combined efforts of the electric heaters and Birgit's rubbing. She dressed me and I positioned myself in a swivel chair to dry out the remaining dampness in my hair. Birgit went to the cooker to turn on the gas under the huge pan of porridge that she'd prepared while I was out running. She'd laid the table, unloaded the dish-washer and got the eggs, bacon and tomatoes all ready for frying.

Facing me across the corner of the table, Birgit edged the large tablespoon round the side of the enormous bowl to collect a mixture of porridge, brown sugar, honey and ice-cream. I swallowed the first delicious spoonful.

'Not too hot?'

'No,' I answered.

'I had a wonderful weekend. We went to the boat and guess what? I steered it under a bridge. It was fantastic! Mr Hawkins showed me how to check the engine-cooling system. The children came to stay. It was cold, but you know how we Swedes like the cold . . .'

While recalling her weekend, Birgit varied the amounts on the spoon and the rate of delivery in response to the subtlest of twitches and grimaces from me.

Throughout her story, unless I heard a particularly arousing word such as 'you', I focused my attention on speculating about further aspects of the illness or pondering the day's commitments.

'I found this decorator. He's going to be great. He only lives down the road. He's going to do a perfect job on the hall, sanding down the woodwork and filling in all the cracks in the walls.'

'You have to watch out for fire on a boat.'

'And he's promised to finish it within a week. What should I pay him per hour? No you don't have to answer. Why should you be interested? Just ignore me. You don't have to listen when I go on like this. My friend from California is flying in. We are going to spend the day in London together.'

'It depends.'

By the time she had cleared the porridge dish away, she had completed her round-up of news. I had run through the different ways a body might adapt to changes in temperature, whether it be the weather, exercise or emotional arousal. Now that my lips and throat were freed from eating, I took the opportunity to make up for my lack of conversation.

'I don't know how much you should pay the decorator. Ask somebody whom he's worked for already and find out how good he is.'

'Do you want two eggs or three?'

'Just two today.'

'Oh! You usually have three.'

'I know, but I'm cutting down on cholesterol. I've just read another report . . .'

'I know all about those reports. You need fattening up.'

'Yes, but not with eggs, which are high in cholesterol.'

'You're not going to cut down on bacon as well, are you?'

'Sorry, yes. Just two rashers, please.'

'But it is so difficult to scramble two eggs. You need at least three.'

'Do your best, Birgit.'

For a number of months Birgit had been trying to maintain a strict diet, which meant she didn't eat any breakfast herself but liked feeding me up. This made me think half the enjoyment of eating might come from cooking. Certainly Birgit's emotions were invested in the breakfast she prepared me: she loved eating.

'You know, it's not work, it's pleasure coming round here. I love early mornings. None of the others at Crossroads do.' She was referring to the organisation she worked for, designed to provide relief for those bogged down caring for handicapped people. Birgit came for two hours, three mornings a week.

'It's terrific that you come. It's a lovely boost. It's sheer luxury having you here.'

'I mean it when I say I like to come. But I don't like too many nights with the others.'

'How many different people have you got?'

'At the moment I've got you, one other with Parkinson's and two with MS.'

A carefully arranged plate of bacon, eggs, tomatoes and half a slice of toast was placed before me. Birgit didn't just provide relief for Jan; she encouraged me to indulge in extravagant meals. I didn't resist. Before she had a chance to fork the first abundant mouthful, I asked her, 'Why do you do Crossroads?'

She told me her husband had died eighteen months before and left her financially well provided for. Two of her three children were still at school and she didn't want a full-time job.

'It was meant to be. I got this job in Bulgaria. I was having an awful time trying to get people interested in me at my age, even though I am a fully qualified nurse. Then while I was on holiday on the Black Sea I met someone who told me about Crossroads and God somehow directed me into joining.'

I turned my head away from the next forkful. I wanted to know why she'd kept it up. Crossroads is not voluntary but its workers get paid only a low hourly rate. She was extremely reliable and sensitive and everything usually went without a hitch.

'I only do it because I want to. I enjoy it. None of that duty nonsense. If I stopped enjoying it, I'd stop doing it. I wouldn't do it if I didn't get paid . . . Yes, I would. I just enjoy . . . well no, sometimes I don't . . . Mmm.'

I tried to draw her into discussing morality and my view that it is not to be identified with doing an altruistic act, perhaps involving a degree of self-sacrifice. Rather it resides in the effort to reconcile what a person thinks ought to be done with his emotions and feelings so that he feels like seeing to it that it is done. But my speech let me down and I got stuck in the mechanics of getting the words out.

I was fascinated by the way she gave herself instructions out loud when she was tired. This sometimes became a running commentary on her thoughts. She got upset if any food fell off the fork or spoon and would go through a variety of defensive ploys: 'It's not much, I'll deal with it later. It wasn't my fault. Perhaps there was too much on the fork.'

After a short interval of silence I said, 'I won't be a minute,' stood up and walked over to the body-dryer. There was a patch of damp hair at the back of my head. It only took a minute to dry out and I was soon back in my chair.

'You are in a good state. Why should that be? I know, you've been taking your drugs.'

I wanted to tell her that it was not quite as simple as that.

'I know you don't like taking them, but I'm sure if you took more you'd be a lot better.'

'As I've explained before . . .'

'You need to put on more weight.'

'But I'm . . .'

'Why don't you have sausages as well?'

'. . . over twelve stone . . . side-effects!'

'Yes, I know all about the side-effects. No I don't. You know better than me.'

I blurted out disjointed phrases reminding her of the unpleasant reactions when I increased the amount of drugs; she agreed they were important and should be taken into account.

After we had got to the toast and jam she said that, in her view, your health was the most important thing in life: if you lost good health, life was not worth living. Fortunately my reaction was too slow to be linked with what she'd said, otherwise I would have been subjected to an embarrassing and tortuous qualification arguing that she did not regard me as having poor health – a view I held too!

Things were beginning to stir upstairs and, fully appreciating the preference of the rest of the family to have breakfast in peace, Birgit started to collect her things together. She gave a cheery goodbye and, like one of the elf cobblers in the Grimms' fairy tale, was suddenly gone, leaving behind not a pile of mended shoes but a well-fed client and a beautifully tidy kitchen. As she was closing the door she said, 'You'd be much better if you took more drugs.'

Experiments at Hull

Ken Flowers had taken up the challenge I'd thrown down at the Eastern Motor Group Meeting and I arranged to spend two days doing some of his experiments at Hull University. My friend Steve came to help and we arranged to stay in my in-laws' house while they were on holiday.

We met Ken at his office in a large suburban house near his department. The weather was balmy and I was feeling relaxed and fluent despite having come off the drugs for the first day of experiments. Ken was very welcoming. We planned to do his standard battery of tests while I was off the drugs and relying on storage from the previous day, and then to repeat the tests the following day with me back on the drugs.

'I thought we'd start with the Webster score to see what state you're in.'

'I've done that before. It's highly subjective and in any case is only relevant to the moment it's taken,' I argued. 'I may be completely unable to perform a particular action, then later, because I've been able to dissipate arousal with some ritual, I get control. Conversely, I may be able to retain control in my arms and hands by using resources for posture and this strategy can then suddenly break down when the resources are used up.'

'Yes,' said Ken, 'but since the score takes into account posture, gait and speech, as well as tremor, rigidity and slowness of movement, to produce a composite measure, this reallocation of resources is allowed for. So if you are achieving dexterity through sacrificing posture and speech, then the combined score would take this into account.'

'I think it's a load of rubbish. It doesn't take account of all the environmental factors that influence control, or lack of it, such as the weather or the interaction of the drugs with food.'

'Yes, I wanted to ask you about that. You are obviously feeling good with this warm weather – presumably fluency fades with cold?'

'Yes, very much. But it's not as simple as that, because even when I'm cold there are periods of fluency.'

'What about tiredness?'

'It depends. The main factor seems to be my emotional state, particularly whether I'm nervous or angry. The higher the level of emotional arousal, the more difficult it is to maintain control. I can try holding the tremor, but this produces rigidity. In fact, I see rigidity as held tremor.'

'Does alcohol help?'

'There is a temporary calming, but greater deficit after a couple of hours.'

'That's the normal reaction, of course!'

'To dissipate tremor I have to try and lower my state of emotional arousal. To get to sleep I have to suppress arousing thoughts.'

'You see tremor as a sign of stress? In that case, are you able to hide your feelings?'

'If I start shaking and can't speak it's a fairly obvious giveaway. I can disguise emotion by holding but I may then go completely rigid!'

'Do you have difficulty getting in and out of bed or chairs?'

'During the course of the day I will be in and out of control because I am reluctant to overlap the doses of drugs, so my capacity to get up varies throughout the day. The problem with being off the drugs is that I can't even hold a book, or I would stay off more. On the drugs all sorts of possibilities bombard consciousness and my thought is much more erratic. As long as there is no time deadline, I anticipate that I will form a better 'mental set', or be able to follow a set of rules, more easily off the drugs than on. If there is a time penalty, tremor will break out, I will forget the instruction, tremor will increase and I will have to use quite extraordinary manoeuvres to regain emotional equilibrium.'

'How about turning over in bed?'

'I rarely do. I lie on my right side. Sleeping position needs to be researched. If I sleep on my back, I may get a good sleep, but all storage will be dissipated by the morning and I will feel dreadful.'

'What about manual dexterity – dressing and using tools, for example, or threading a needle?'

'Yes, in this state I would have great difficulty. But you must not just differentiate between the "on" and "off" states. The longer I stay off, the worse I get.'

'What about memory?'

'I believe the problem with Parkinson's is one of retrieval and not memory storage. I can test whether the drug is wearing off by trying to remember the names of the heads of department at college. My success rate and the time it takes me relate directly to the level of transmitter available. I use mnemonic devices to provide an alternative, non-emotional coding. The sillier the better. I use the visual mnemonic of a gang of hooligans playing a double bass to remember "basal ganglia".'

'I'd like to try a memory test of verbal learning. I am going to read a list of fifteen words and see how many you can remember. We will repeat the test until you can remember all fifteen and see how many goes it takes you.'

We did a number of other tests and then, in the afternoon, went over to the department to do a series of tests of motor control. Steve took me to the loo, choosing the sunny cubicle on the end. He dropped my pants and lowered me on to the seat. We started giggling as someone else came in and my tremor made the thin walls of the partition reverberate. The person made a rapid exit!

We were shown into the lab and met Ken's two colleagues. I was sat in a chair facing a screen, surrounded by oscilloscopes, computer printers and other paraphernalia. They asked me to take off my T-shirt so that they could fix electrodes to my shoulders, but the chap fixing them kept treading on the wires and pulling them off. The oscilloscope refused to work properly.

'Do you find yourselves doing experiments the computer likes, rather than things you want to do?' I asked.

'There's always problems with equipment. The more complex the apparatus, the greater the chance of something going wrong,' said Ken. 'But we can start now. You've done this sort of thing before in London. A target of two parallel lines will appear on the screen, then a dot. The task is to control the dot with the lever in front of you and move it to within the target as quickly as possible.'

'Is this well stuck down!' I exclaimed, as my shaking hand gripped the lever. 'Can I rest between trials?'

'Yes. If you push the lever forwards, the computer will delay presenting the next target without any penalty.'

'Then it'll be dead easy!' I said. 'The rest periods will be critical in allowing me to dissipate the rigidity which will build up from holding back the tremor.'

I sat hunched over the lever, my face reflected in the blank screen – a wide-eyed hawk, hook nose and glaring eyes, talons clamping the lever in a vice-like grip, hovering over the screen waiting for the dot to appear so that I could swoop.

'I'm over-shooting the small targets close to the bottom of the screen which need very small, precise movements.'

'We have found that all the people with Parkinson's we have tested have this problem. They have difficulty making use of prior information to control movement. Normal people are much quicker if they are able to anticipate the position and size of the target from the previous series.'

'You need to repeat the test at the same time tomorrow to take account of the biological rhythms affecting arousal and control,' I said. 'My left hand seems less susceptible to self-conscious arousal than my right. I was much calmer during the practice period when it was playful and didn't matter.'

After two or three hours we went back to Ken's office.

'The final experiment I want to try is to test your ability to follow a mental rule. I am going to show you cards with four letters on them, three of which are the same and one different, some in upper case, some in lower case, some in outline, others solid. Say which is the odd one out.'

I did as he asked.

'Now we'll go through them again,' he said, 'but using a different rule.'

We went through the cards eight times. I found it boring, but was reluctant to be counted among the dunces.

'How do people with Parkinson's compare with the norm?'

'People without Parkinson's make random errors flipping from one rule to another, which they check and then correct. Parkinson's patients seem unable to switch rules once embarked on a sequence. They have much less difficulty if the same rule is maintained rather than alternated. You don't seem to have had much trouble.'

'I'm able to overcome the deficit at this level of storage, but I would be unable to if I stayed off the drug much longer. I want to be really stretched with these tests. I don't think I'm being taxed sufficiently really to demonstrate the deficit of Parkinson's.'

'See how you get on with this test of digit span.'

I did less well remembering numbers than words. I found I could remember a sequence of numbers in reverse.

'Breaking up the order can be beneficial to short-term memory for people with Parkinson's,' Ken said.

'I'm having to give up the basic need for postural control to achieve the task. The deeper and deeper I go into deficit, the nearer I get to a catastrophic threshold beyond which I am totally unable to act.'

We returned the following morning after a good night's sleep. I had taken my usual dose of drugs and felt good. Ken repeated his Webster assessment. I returned to the attack.

'It's all very well you scoring me high. I can get out of the chair and walk around fluently, but I can't do other important things. There are other aspects of performance, such as thinking, which you aren't measuring. It's crazy to do experiments with people on the drugs; they wipe out the Parkinson deficit.'

'The drugs ameliorate the symptoms, they don't eliminate the condition,' said Ken.

'On the drug, with dyskinesia, it's like being pushed around by the drug. You can't regulate the excess.'

'That's like a behavioural description of fatigue.'

'I can relax with the tremor and achieve a kind of stillness. With the drugs, the initial state of normality quickly passes into writhing. It's so difficult to gauge the body's rate of absorption of the drug. They have tried an infusion system, but the acidity of the L-dopa entering the bloodstream directly causes problems and the drug has to be diluted.'

'But you are on the drugs now. You're in control, your voice is strong, you can move fluently. Isn't this a much better state than yesterday when you were off the drugs?'

'Yes. The Parkinson deficit is totally eliminated.'

'Then what's wrong?'

'I'm not saying that being on the drug, even with the side-effects of dyskinesia, is worse or that people are daft for taking the drugs. But, given my personality, I prefer the non-drug state. In a strange way I feel more in control, even though I have less control in a motor sense. There are motor problems on the drugs. The dyskinesia pushes you. My shoulder jerks when I write and I have to reschedule the writhing in a similar way as the tremor.'

'Try writing now.'

'I am able to write by curling my toes and gripping the carpet. The writhing finds expression within the elements of the writing. I can use it to form the letters. When I'm off the drugs I can control tremor too but, after holding it back, it always breaks out later in wilder shaking or rigidity. In contrast, the dyskinesia on the drugs finds expression in the action and is dissipated. The dyskinesia produces a behavioural interference rather than the deeper undermining of control that the tremor entails.'

'I give you a Webster score of two today, compared with ten yesterday. A score of nought is normal and twenty the maximum Parkinson deficit,' said Ken. I decided not to argue and we repeated the memory tests.

'Off the drugs I can slowly wind my way methodically over an area of memory. My mode of thinking off the drugs and relying on storage is analytical. On the drugs, with concurrent dopamine slushing around in my nervous system, my brain overactively makes connections, one idea overlaying another.'

'It's similar to the over-arousal of mania when too much is generated?'

'It's different – the arousal of mania produces chaos. The drugs allow a viable synthesis. I can just dip into the chaos and pull out the gems. It feels highly creative. The most creative phase is when the drugs have reached the brain and become available as dopamine but have not yet been induced to serve muscular motor function. The problem is one of holding on to the ideas and connections until I'm in a position to record them. If I take a high dose of drugs there may be enough to serve both the control of muscle and the operation of memory and creative thought. But there's a huge risk of severe unwanted writhing movement.'

'Is thought itself slower off the drugs?'

'Yes. I think there is an upward inhibitory effect from lack of motor control which dampens down cortical activity to cope with the motor disability. However, this may not occur for some time, owing to the benefits of storage. Maybe only a particular kind of thought is affected – that geared to action. Perhaps abstract thought and fantasy are unaffected.'

'There seems to be strong evidence that people with Parkinson's disease make more errors and have more difficulty planning the sequencing of action than normal people. It would seem that high-level planning functions are impaired.'

'Yes. A good example of that is getting my breakfast. I have to fetch the elements that form the breakfast – the milk, sugar, spoon – one at a time. It is hard to co-ordinate a sequence of action, and having to speak to someone in the middle can totally undermine the action. In contrast, when I've taken the drug the bombardment of thoughts can interfere with holding on to a simple plan. There is no motor difficulty co-ordinating actions but I can get stuck deciding whether to wash the dishes or lay the table! When off the drug, the barely possible action gets disrupted through interference from seeing, hearing or thinking of something different; on the drug a host of actions become possible and failure to keep to a particular action is through being spoilt for choice. Off the drug one is struggling to hold out against disruption of the sequence of component elements of a single action; by taking the drug the problem becomes one of holding out against interruption from an attraction towards numerous other quite feasible acts.'

'That's what happens in the rules' test.'

'For variety I'm going to try a different rule to yesterday,' I said.

We repeated the test with the lettered cards eight times and Ken smilingly announced that I was no worse today than yesterday.

I had assumed I would have performed better the previous day, off the drugs. Ken's stance of testing patients on their drugs was substantiated. I was surprised. I shouldn't have been, though, because the states one goes through are more complex than simply being 'on' or 'off' the drugs and the tests hadn't really stretched me.

We went over to the university staff canteen for lunch and had suet-crusted steak-and-kidney pudding. I felt more and more uncomfortable, and Steve said, 'You look very pale – are you all right?'

I raced for the loo and disgorged the lunch.

'That's another problem with the drugs. They can induce nausea if they interact in the wrong way with food.'

'Yes, it was very salty. Are you going to be able to repeat the lever test?'

'Yes, I'll be fine in a minute.'

This time I did the test much faster and was probably just as accurate. I noticed my reflection in the screen. I was leaning back in the chair, head tipped back and skewed round. I felt relaxed and confident and held the joystick lightly between fingers and thumb like a hot-shot pilot.

'I'm in a very good state for this. I'm adopting a much riskier strategy: swooping in fast as soon as the dot appears and slowing down to lock on to the target.'

We had tea and set off back to Cambridge that afternoon, with Ken's good wishes for a safe journey.

I felt that the trip had been worthwhile. Although the tests hadn't shown what I expected, I thought I had successfully argued that it was of limited use to compare Parkinson patients on a full drug regime with subjects who didn't have the disease. I felt I had gone some way to convincing Ken of the value of testing patients like me who were experimenting with their drug management.

Out of Control in Marks and Spencer

The symbol for the disabled appears throughout Marks and Spencer along with the words 'Happy to Help'. I never expected to take up this offer, but it was comforting all the same. I had Justin to drive me into town when he was free. If I got into difficulties I could get back to the car and either wait for control to be restored so that I could make another foray to complete my shopping, or be driven home straightaway.

On one memorable trip the weather was dreadful and the windscreen wipers could hardly work fast enough to maintain visibility. We found a parking space a short distance from the rear entrance to the store. Jus asked if I wanted him to come round the shop with me, but I said no; we decided each to do our own shopping and meet back at the car in three-quarters of an hour. I didn't expect to take anything like that long and thought I would have to wait in the car for Jus to return.

In the store, I decided to leave buying the food till the end, so I walked straight across to the escalator. I felt in good form and consciously reassured myself that the drugs would hold out. I saw a friend called Morag on the down escalator but couldn't afford to get delayed in conversation. On the way round to the next flight I caught sight of someone else I knew with a grey beard going in the other direction. He looks rough, I thought, as I looked away.

I left the escalator and started the hunt for Shetland wool pullovers. I was aware of a vague feeling of familiarity and pretty soon the quick flashes of recognition I was experiencing as I moved around were suddenly filled with meaning. Narrow vertical mirrors were fixed to all the pillars. I stopped to look at my reflection. I saw a tall, angular body, slightly stooped, with a neck that seemed to snake a path through the air, and wide, staring eyes. The remaining tufts of fast-thinning hair were plastered to my head. I made a feeble attempt to improve the appearance of this unattractive figure by dragging my fingers through my hair.

I couldn't just stand there doing myself up, though. I moved to a different stack of clothes and snatched glances at myself in another mirror. I was shocked by the amount of head movement produced by the marionette-like reflection. However much I tried to put a favourable interpretation on what I'd seen, it was impossible to get away from the constant reminders from these mirrored pillars.

I found the colour and size of pullover that I wanted and stood in the queue to pay. A woman in front was insisting on having the cashier swap a pair of trousers one size larger than the pair she had bought the previous day and was now returning. The cashier was trying to explain that the place for exchanges was in another part of the store with the carefully chosen neutral title of 'Customer Services'. I did my best to shut out the excited undercurrent to the exchange; I was feeling considerable strain and just wanted to pay for my pully and get on the escalator back down.

Although the assistant was very young, she seemed to appreciate that I would benefit from an encouraging and friendly manner. Having run the gauntlet of the mirrors, the escalator's steady slowness gave me a chance to compose myself. My confidence was diminished and I felt uncertain about my control. Nevertheless, I decided to buy the food. There were hardly any queues at the checkouts.

There were eight things I had to buy. I didn't like having to carry lists and recalled the mnemonic that I had constructed from the first letter of each item: 'stumclip'. I hurried as fast as possible, filling my basket with lettuce, pears, ice-cream, unbroken biscuits . . . and then I was stuck. The contents of the basket began to rattle and bounce. I was mad with myself for not heeding the early warnings. I chose a place near the freezers to put the basket down on the floor where it was least likely to get in people's way.

I decided to carry on and complete the list. I was fed up with having to break off tasks half completed. I succeeded in getting the tomatoes. I had to pitch the mince pies on to a shelf of chicken legs before resuming the journey and dropping them into the basket. The Stilton was not in its usual place, so I abandoned it. I had forgotten that Marks didn't do cider. By now I was in a bad way.

I toyed with the idea of asking an assistant if she could carry my basket to be checked out. But how would I get the stuff to the car? I needed both hands free to clasp each other behind my back to save myself from falling forwards, but I couldn't really expect anyone to walk all the way to the car in the pouring rain. So I yanked the pullover from the bottom of the basket and jammed it into the top of my trousers, leaving my hands free. I must have provided a spectacle to the people round me as I shook the wrapping paper almost to tearing point.

I abandoned the basket of food for the time being, placing it to one side next to the drinks section. The idea was to go back to the car, take some more drugs and try to come back after twenty minutes or so. It was still raining heavily. I ran, fell, stumbled and slid my way to the car. All the doors were locked: I had forgotten to remind Jus not to lock the one on my side. The rain was pouring down my face and I could hardly see through my glasses. I stood leaning against the car with one hand grasping the roof-rack, the other tapping violently against the door. I had the idea of taking refuge in a nearby church . . . they always used to be open, but nowadays you could never tell. I thought about a shop entrance, but there would be nothing to hold on to. So I stayed where I was.

After twenty minutes Jusie came back. As he saw me he exclaimed, 'What! Can't you get in? Oh, I'm sorry, Dad.'

Completely soaked, with water running down my neck, I assured him that it was all right. He opened the door and I collapsed in an uncomfortable heap on the seat. I thought of telling him about the food but couldn't face the effort of a long explanation of where he might find the basket. He started the car and we drove home. As we were getting out he looked round for the shopping to carry it into the house.

'Where's the food, Dad?'

'I didn't manage to buy it, Jus. The things weren't urgent anyway.'

Martham Diet

We couldn't find Pat's house, 'Moonriver', so Erick, with whom she ran a sailing school, came and met us on the green in Martham, in Norfolk, and took us to the riverside chalet where I was to spend a week on Pat's diet. That evening, over an excellent meal, she explained her approach of banning a whole range of foods and then reintroducing them one by one. In this way she had discovered that gluten, dairy products and red meat produced allergic reactions and by cutting them from her diet had been able to reduce the crippling symptoms of her arthritis. She had suffered acutely with arthritis since childhood, but after twenty years had finally made a breakthrough.

I was highly sceptical about the possibility of diet influencing the actual progress of Parkinson's disease but thought that there might be an interaction effect on the drugs and the severity of the symptoms. I had already stopped drinking tea because intuitively I felt it caused hypertension during the night.

Pat Byrivers had written to me after the *Horizon* programme and we had arranged that I should spend a week at one of her riverside bungalows on the Broads. Steve and his wife, Scharlie, drove me there but could only stay for the first part of the week. I didn't hesitate to turn this to my advantage, as I felt it would be a challenge to cope on my own for the three days before Steve came to collect me, and Pat and Erick would be on hand to help in emergencies.

We were impressed by Pat's ease of movement, which substantiated the treatment methods discussed in her recently published book, *Goodbye to Arthritis*. Over dinner we found both her and Erick enjoyable company and looked forward to being taken sailing the next day. Pat had written asking if there was anything special I was likely to need. I was in a good state of control when I replied that there was nothing. As usual, I found it difficult to envisage the difficulties I might experience. Those I did manage to remember were quickly glossed over.

Our first taste of the diet when we arrived – gluten-free biscuits and a drink of warm water – was somewhat Spartan, but the evening meal of green vegetables, baked potatoes and a small portion of chicken, followed by fruit and soya custard, was entirely acceptable.

As Steve pulled the blanket into place over me that night I didn't mention that I might not be able to get comfortable on the soft mattress. My feet edged their way down the bed and far too soon they touched the iron rail that marked the end of the mattress. This would mean strain at both ends of my body, my ankles holding my feet and my neck holding my head. However, I was still confident.

I hadn't brought a clock so I couldn't tell whether the little light that filtered through the curtains was dawn or just moonlight. If it was only about two o'clock, then it was pointless letting myself wake up further through the urge to go for a pee because I wouldn't be able to get out of bed. I was daft not to have brought a clock, but without my glasses I couldn't see the time and, anyway, I wouldn't have been able to control the tremor long enough to lift the clock. I needed a miniature church with dead quiet chimes.

Would the chemical loo move if the tremor became very strong? What if I tipped it over? My imagination ran riot with images of myself crawling on the floor splattered with sludge, flesh burning and throat choking from the navy-blue chemical. The only thing to do was to lie and wait for the morning boost of fluency. All heaviness had gone from my eyes as they darted around the almost black room. I was stupid to allow myself to imagine such vivid and arousing scenes when I knew I couldn't cope with them. The mantra allowed me to get fairly calm again, but it didn't last for long and the knocking, tapping and rattling started anew. Surely Steve and Scharlie in the next room would be having a terrible night.

About an hour and a half passed before the morning's major surge in fluency. It was fairly weak, but sufficient to give me the idea of peeing in the wash-basin instead of the loo out in the garden. The light-switch in the bedroom was broken; I spent five minutes getting it to work. I stopped myself blaming Pat and Erick. It was still dark when I fell back on to the bed.

I felt a mixture of pleasure and foreboding when Steve came out of his room next morning at about half past eight. I was convinced that they could have hardly slept at all.

'I won't ask you if you've had a bad night. I'm very sorry.'

'What do you mean? We slept perfectly. I heard you tapping, but then I went straight back to sleep.'

'Come off it!'

'Well, I can't speak for Scharlie, but I'm sure she slept as well as I did.'

'That's incredible.'

Sitting like a couple of ancient seafarers with our cushions and blankets on the wooden bench in front of the chalet, we could survey a wide stretch of the River Thurn with its passing boats and its wildlife. Faced by a curtain of reeds, the tuck-box of permitted goodies in front of us, we sat there talking. I was soon forced to remove my glasses to cut out the variety of interesting but interrupting events going on around me and, more importantly, to block out the reactions of people as they noticed me. The trouble was that if I heard something interesting, I couldn't check to see what it was and I would spin off into a round of wondering and distraction. However, I wasn't so shortsighted that I could avoid noticing the struggling engine of the old wooden slop-out boat as two men arrived to empty the latrine. And I put my glasses back on to appreciate the silent grace of the brown-sailed wherry, under full sail, its mast stretching forty feet above the water as it creamed past, dominating the river.

As the morning passed, it needed more and more effort to trade off muscle control for enhanced generation and retrieval of ideas. My voice grew increasingly inaudible, words were slurred together and pressure to economise made me pass over longer words and go for short ones even at cost to the sense of what I was saying.

Two yachts were moored alongside the chalet, and later that day Pat and Erick invited us to go for a sail. (Erick Manners was a yacht designer, world-famous for his revolutionary catamarans and trimarans.) It was Steve and Scharlie's first time sailing but, with expert tuition, they were soon practising quite complicated manoeuvres.

As we sneaked along the narrow channel to Horsham Broad, I frequently checked the river for signs of the wherry's huge bulk. It would be interesting to see how we'd get past if the wind made it necessary to tack. Once in the Broad, the change from the constricting channel to the freedom of wide open space was accompanied by a lessening of tension. It was like the feeling I often have when locked in the queue at Sainsbury's checkout – there comes a moment of relief when the banker's card is handed back and I push the trolley through the automatic doors into the car park.

However, the sense of freedom was spoilt somewhat by a hint of nausea. I had taken some extra drugs but seemed to have misjudged it. If I lay down, I knew I could stop it, but I didn't want to disturb the others' pleasure. It was a beautiful day, and Erick and Pat were clearly very happy to see their visitors having a good time. The wind got up, the boat heeled to forty-five degrees and the flow of exhilaration matched the rush of water through my fingers. The pallor of my face gave the game away.

'Are you all right? You've been looking very pale.' I hadn't altogether succeeded in freeing Steve from the role of looking after me. Clearly he couldn't break the habit of checking periodically to see if I was all right.

'I'm afraid I feel a bit sick,' I confessed. I knew I'd gone past the point where it would subside. Steve had intuitively delayed asking, realising that this risked interrupting one of the coping strategies. I moved into position, neck stretched out over the water.

'I'll be all right.' I felt somebody grip the straps of my life-jacket. I emptied my stomach in a series of barks and honks. On the few occasions when I was sick there was always a brief explosion followed by a good feeling of control and relaxation. I was able to reassure everybody that I was fine and made it clear that it wasn't necessary to go back sooner than planned. I must have convinced them, because we continued criss-crossing the Broad for another half-hour before returning to the narrow channel. Erick offered me a turn at the tiller as we tacked our way back home, but my limbs had passed out of control and begun to shake.

It is a strange kind of nausea. Within a very short time I was ready to eat, fully confident I would not be sick again. Perhaps it is because the nausea is initiated by chemicals in the brain, rather than by something that is eaten or drunk. As soon as we went indoors I was looking forward to the meal. Pat had provided a tuck-box of between-meal snacks: nuts, sweetmeats, carob bars of sesame seed, and peanut brittle. I went at these as if entering the gorging phase of the anorexic cycle. An hour later we were round the table for the evening meal.

'What would you like to drink? There's fruit juice for everybody except Ivan. He can have warm water.'

We all laughed and I was quick to point out that I had already discovered I could drink warm water as a substitute for tea and coffee. I'd come to Martham ready to put up with little else besides bread and water, as this was supposed to be an elimination diet, although I don't know how long I would have lasted after eating the rather tasteless crumbly bread!

Pat had decided to concentrate on eliminating gluten and animal fat. Porridge was out! A huge range of things were forbidden but the bread was made more palatable through a spread of honey or ginger jelly. Pat proved that a credible diet with a wide variety of dishes was possible. On this occasion she served rice salad, green salad, potatoes, carrots and green beans.

'You can have as many vegetables as you like,' she said, as I ladled masses of rice on to my plate. For pudding there was a choice of bananas, pears, mango or peaches, which Pat said were non-acidic and agreed with most people. I tipped a whole carton of soya custard on to a bowl of peaches. To finish, I chewed my way through half a bag of figs followed by a couple of fistfuls of Brazil nuts.

While Steve reorganised my mattress on the floor in the living room to prevent a repeat of the previous night, I filled out a questionnaire Pat had devised to check any change from day to day. I had been highly critical of an enquiry into depression and Parkinson's carried out a couple of years previously by a professional scientific researcher. He had failed to draw important distinctions between circumstances likely to affect the results. In Pat's case, it would be pointless to raise objections of that kind as we were looking for major changes in the pattern of daily behaviour.

After Scharlie and Steve had left, the routine of the remaining few days was quickly established: up at seven, an attempt on the loo, a walk, and bread and honey which I was able to eat by means of a spoon, fork and fingers. Pat came in at nine and fed me the rest of my breakfast – Rice Crispies bathed in Coffeemate, with honey as a sweetener. I was then left to read the paper. By taking drugs around eleven, I was able to feed myself lunch. In the afternoon we either went to the shops or for a sail. After supper we'd chat for a bit, then I'd either read or watch television before falling into bed.

The quality of my sleep varied, but on the Thursday night it was a disaster. For a couple of weeks my ears had been blocked, so I didn't hear the high-pitched whining of the mosquito until the last moment as it dropped down on the warmth of my face. I froze with shock and with the thought that, since the whine had stopped, I was being eaten. An attempt to brush my hand across my face made me shake violently.

I tugged on the blanket, which was tucked under one side of the mattress to prevent me getting tangled. Now I desperately wanted some surplus blanket to protect my face from the insect's bombardments. The more I panicked, the hotter I became and the more attractive I was to the mosquito, as the blood flooded the channels near the surface of the skin to cool my body temperature. With a mighty effort I shifted the blanket sufficiently to enable me to make a kind of igloo-tunnel in front of my face, which would allow me to breathe fresh air but would, hopefully, discourage further attack. All my senses were on full alert, my ears straining to hear.

I listened intently and knew that as long as the breaks in the whining were very short the mosquito was landing on the blanket and flying off again in its search for exposed flesh. I decided to push my hand out into the open as a sacrifice, hoping that it would be satisfied and go away.

There was no hope of relaxing sufficiently to trip into sleep. I lay there awake for most of the night, eyes blinking in the dark, blindly tracking the mosquito's progress above me. Next morning I emerged exhausted, but fortunately without having been too much devoured.

There were no effects from change in the diet and no noticeable effects when I returned to my regular foods. It had been a long shot, since nowhere in the literature had there been any reports of gluten or animal fats either causing Parkinson's in the first place or exacerbating the symptoms once the illness had developed.

Ideally, I would have stopped taking my medication for a couple of days to see if without it the absence of gluten and animal fat would arrest the deterioration of my condition, but Pat and Erick were quite happy to note if any improvement occurred while I continued taking the drugs. The final check was made when I got home and checked whether there was an adverse reaction after I resumed my normal diet: gluten first, then animal fat the following day.

I rang Pat to give her the disappointing news that I couldn't feel any change. I emphasised to her my view that our mini-investigation should not be used as a justification for not enquiring further into the effect of diet on Parkinson's. In fact, no conclusions whatsoever could be drawn. The diet should be regarded simply as an exploratory exercise, in the hope that ideas for more rigorous experimentation might arise from it.

Hard Drugs

A friend sent me a cutting from *New Scientist* entitled 'Heroin Contaminant Offers Clues to Parkinson's Disease'. The article related that doctors in the USA had begun combing northern California for young heroin addicts who might have injected a contaminated drug that 'caused' Parkinson's. This was a real breakthrough. Up until then the disease had been without a known cause.

The link between a bad batch of synthetic heroin and Parkinsonism was established in 1983 when an addict was admitted to the Santa Clara Valley Medical Center, run by William Langston. After some quite incredible medical detective work, the doctors concluded that the addict was the victim of a 'designer-drug disaster'. Instead of injecting himself with synthetic heroin, he had used a contaminant known as MPTP. This had set off in his brain a chemical reaction that had induced damage to the *substantia nigra*, that group of cells implicated in Parkinson's disease.

The article went on to say:

Little is known about the progression of Parkinsonism in an individual because often the elderly people who are stricken die of other causes.

It is possible that a single incident – in this case the contaminated drug – sets in motion a series of events that shows up years later as a degenerative disease.

Langston and others believe that chemicals in the environment – even MPTP – are the cause of Parkinsonism in the general population.

An American friend with Parkinson's disease gave a copy of my *Listener* article to Dr Langston, who sent me two of his articles and a very encouraging letter. In one of these articles he wrote:

Based on currently available evidence, one can launch a formidable argument that Parkinson's disease is due to an environmental toxin.

First, the completion of a twin study of Parkinson's disease (Ward,

1983) has provided strong evidence against a purely genetic origin for the disease. The concordance rate among twins, in which at least one twin had typical Parkinson's disease, was very low.

If not genetic in origin, then the disease must be due to something in the environment, but what? The two most obvious candidates are infectious agents and toxins.

In regard to infectious agents . . . Parkinson's disease is virtually devoid of the neuropathological hallmarks of an infectious process. Finally, the disease has yet to prove transmissible. This line of reasoning leaves us with an environmental toxin as the major remaining contender.

Progess was being made not only with the aetiology of the disease but also in its treatment.

In spite of Langston's evidence and arguments, I doubted that the cause was always attributable to the environment. I was finding it very difficult to give up my hypothesis based upon stress. It could accommodate a wide range of circumstances – chronic fever, phobias, exposures to extremes of temperature, prolonged childbirth, continuous participation in high-risk activities – that may entail a breakdown of coping on the part of those brain cells whose destruction or exhaustion eventually results in the symptoms of Parkinson's disease.

John Williams had been the first to tell me about a new drug, selegiline, which was taken alongside L-dopa and which prevented the destruction of dopamine in the brain. Just as Carbidopa helped to stop L-dopa from being destroyed outside the brain, so this new drug conserved the dopamine after it had been synthesised in the brain.

I found it puzzling that the drug selegiline, marketed as Eldepryl and Deprenyl, had been available for over a decade in some countries. Why had it taken so long for research centres to test the ideas of people like Birkmayer in view of the importance of what they were claiming?

John wrote to me in exasperation at the unwillingness I had expressed to try the new drug from which he was deriving such benefit, and offered to let me have a few of his pills. I had been completely ignoring my principle of openness. Here was someone who'd had Parkinson's for almost as long as myself, who was managing the drug-taking extremely successfully and, if I was prepared to admit it, far better than I was. I decided I had to try it out.

Some of the claims made for the drug were exciting, though speculative. One of them was that it slowed down the progress of the disease. Did this mean that for all this time there had been a drug that could have protected me from deterioration had I only known? In my usual way I embarked on a private search for someone or something to blame. Scientists ought to be more willing to acknowledge the role of speculation in the phase of generating the ideas that lead to hypotheses for rigorous scientific testing; journals should encourage them to include accounts of how such ideas arose and were successfully preserved – researchers might then be less likely to ignore the potential of others' ideas on the ground that the way they have been tested is full of flaws. It reminded me of Eysenck's opposition to reports linking smoking with cancer because the level of rigour in the scientific tests did not meet his very high standards.

Recently I had read somewhere about a long-term national study that had been set up to compare three different forms of treatment. It was due to go on for six years. Patients were to be asked if they would like to take part and, if they agreed, they were to be assigned to one of three treatments. One of these was L-dopa combined with a peripheral decarboxylase inhibitor; another was bromocriptine, a stimulator of dopamine nerve receptors; and the third was a combination of the first treatment and Eldepryl.

It seemed to me to be a bit late in the day to be carrying out such an investigation. Patients thinking of taking part in the study should consider asking their doctor what they did in the case of patients who chose to stay out of the study: did they toss a coin as the basis of deciding which of these forms of medication the patient was to have? Or did the doctor have a preference for one of the others? If the patient learned that there *was* a preference, he should check whether this coincided with the treatment which he would have been given had he agreed to take part in the experiments. If they matched, he could stay in the experiment; if they did not, he should withdraw and go for the other treatment which the doctor preferred.

There seemed to me to be a crucial ethical question to be sorted out. If it turned out that one of the treatments was superior, participants who had been given the other treatments would want to be sure that on both experimental and intuitive grounds there had not been a basis for preferring the more successful treatment from which they had been denied a chance to benefit.

The only possible way round the difficulty seemed to be the use of patients who had been diagnosed six years ago and treated with L-dopa plus the inhibitor. They might then be compared six years from now with a sample of patients who were just being started on a treatment recognised as preferable.

Finally, I hoped that each group would be assessed both for the degree to which the symptoms progressed and for how successfully the drugs were helping the patient to cope with everyday life. Would they be looking at any benefit regarding storage?

Before taking the drug, I checked with Professor Marsden whether he thought there was any possibility that it might affect my mood, as it seemed to work in a way similar to anti-depressants, and the last thing I wanted was to become dependent on a daily 'fix' to keep cheerful. I don't suffer from depression – in the most collapsed state imaginable, although my gestures signal utter misery and my speech is reduced to an inaudible mutter, I'm telling the truth when I squeeze out the words, 'I'm feeling very happy.' All the same, if I had to stay in that state I think I would eventually succumb to depression, whatever the particular way in which it is thought to arise. It might seem to be due to a compensatory siphoning off from resources serving mood in order to support more obvious motor functions, or to a spread of the disease mechanism to cells providing resources for sustaining a coping mood or outlook.

I also wanted reassurance that those precious hours in the morning when I benefit from storage wouldn't be lost.

It was eight years after Parkinson's was diagnosed. I was reluctant to admit it, but I was beginning to require very high doses of L-dopa to maintain sufficient levels of storage to go running, shower and feed myself breakfast. In spite of all I've said about not suffering depression, this deterioration was beginning to sadden my outlook, because I didn't want to give up my running and make adjustments to more realistic aspirations.

Professor Marsden wrote back and said that I needn't worry on either of these counts.

I wrote to Iain Wilkinson and told him that I intended to start taking Eldepryl. I already had an appointment fixed with him, but it had been changed by the hospital administration to a date only four days before Jan and I were due to go to Venice on holiday. This was unfortunate, as it would allow insufficient time for me to re-establish my existing regime of L-dopa should the new drug either not work at all or produce strange, unwanted effects. Besides, I wanted to have time to play around with the timing and amount of drug taken. So instead of getting Eldepryl from Iain, I wrote to John to take up his offer and he sent me a week's supply. This would carry me over until my appointment with Iain. And so I began to take Eldepryl.

In my usual way, I found myself unable simply to follow the prescribed pattern of drug-taking designed to keep the symptoms under control twenty-four hours a day. I couldn't resist exploring different approaches, partly because of that intransigent commitment to self-determination and partly in case I hit on a style which reduced the dyskinesias to a significantly greater extent than that claimed by the manufacturers.

The research reports suggested that the new drug made it possible to cut back on L-dopa by about thirty per cent. Its effectiveness was supposed to last up to twelve hours. John was taking it first thing in the morning and again at midday as a boost. On both occasions he combined it with a low dose of L-dopa. To start with, I thought I'd do the same – lowering the amount of L-dopa by about a third.

On the first day of taking the new drug it was difficult to detect any effect in the morning. I managed to get 'on' in spite of the reduction but the fluency didn't last any longer than usual, although Eldepryl was supposed to have an extended period of effectiveness.

In the afternoon, instead of falling asleep as I usually do somewhere between two and four o'clock, I managed to stay awake. I immediately toyed with the idea that this might be due to an amphetamine-like effect. The literature on Eldepryl mentioned that the chemical later metabolised into a weak form of amphetamine and once I'd got hold of that idea I couldn't shake it off.

In the evening, after a large meal, I thought I'd revert to my usual dose of L-dopa to make sure that it would 'take' quickly and have worn off by the time I wanted to go to sleep.

In the middle of the night I woke up in a very tight foetal position, my knees drawn up to my chest and my neck curling round off the pillow. I felt as though I had been very deeply asleep, and now I was completely stuck. I couldn't check the time, but was sure that it wasn't anywhere near four o'clock; it would be a long wait till the early-morning boost. Would it happen at all?

I became aware of my clarity of thought and began to have ambitious notions, such as stretching my legs and moving my right shoulder to a different position. Heightened fluency in my muscles suddenly appeared, and I quickly took advantage of it to check the time in case I became stuck again. It was quarter past two. Extraordinary! The flood of available resources prompted a wide range of even more extravagant projects.

For the rest of the night I enjoyed great clarity of thought as I nimbly hopped from one idea to another in the search to solve fresh puzzles. I waited to see if I would get a 'super boost' or if that had been used up in the fluency achieved earlier. Nothing happened. But downstairs later on, as I was getting my shoes on in preparation for running, I noticed that, although I had considerable tremor, I was assuming an ambitiously long run. I felt confident about meeting other people and looked forward to putting this feeling to the test. I became concerned that the drug might turn me into an over-confident fool.

At lunch the following day I lost fluency as the effects of the first dosage came to an end, yet I managed to feed myself; Jan and I both remarked on the ease with which I did this. I slept much longer in the night, with vivid, highly arousing dreams. There was still sufficient storage for me to make breakfast and shower after a modest run. However, I couldn't contain my curiosity about the effect of administering the drug differently.

I came up with the idea that the breakdown of dopamine may occur particularly during sleep. If that were inhibited in a major way, perhaps storage could be made even better. Accordingly, I took a dose of the new drug immediately before going to bed the next evening. The effect was dramatic – I didn't sleep at all!

I thought I would try the drug at around half past four in the morning to see if it would preserve the benefit of early-morning storage. It would be very useful if I could fall asleep again, confident that the store of dopamine would not be depleted through oxidation caused by a bout of dreaming.

Parkinson's in Venice

We sat wedged into outside seats, our eyes buffeted by a succession of novel sensations, as the water-bus zigzagged from stop to stop along the Grand Canal. The journey lasted forty minutes. The pilot nudged the boat against our landing-stage and I was delighted at how close we were to the Piazza San Marco. We let the other people get off and Jan took out the piece of paper with the Tourist Office instructions for finding our hotel. I persuaded her to put off the search for a few minutes to look back down the canal and appreciate the extraordinary blend of colours in the light of the setting sun, the harmony of heavy and delicate buildings and the gentle movement of swaying gondolas tied to their moorings. The water lapping against the quay created the illusion that we had stepped into a painting by Canaletto.

The thumping of the next ferry as another batch of passengers flowed on to the stone water-front brought us back to the quest for our hotel.

'I think that must be it.' It stood on the other side of a wide marble bridge at the point where one of the city's canals fingered its way into the open lagoon.

We were given the keys to adjoining single rooms on the fourth floor. It wasn't that we didn't have a choice or that we'd had a row on the plane; I'd long since got used to sleeping in a separate bedroom at home because of the racket I made in the night and neither of us wanted to risk sleepless nights when there was so much to do and enjoy.

Jan opened the window and pushed back the shutters. Across a broad stretch of water stood the huge church of San Giorgio Maggiore and by leaning out we could see the lofty tower of San Marco. It was beginning to get dark but we both felt like going out. Straightaway I was struck by the quality of sounds in the traffic-free streets. We could hear the tap of shoes on stone echoing up the steep-sided buildings. At one moment we were walking down a deserted cul-de-sac, then in a couple of turns our way was filled with Italian hubbub.

We walked towards the Rialto bridge, using the map sparingly so that we didn't ruin the pleasure that comes from surprise. The main routes were brightly lit but minor alleyways were dark and mediaeval. We whispered aloud the names of the elegant squares and impressive buildings as we walked: 'Palazzo Grassi', 'Campo Santa Sophia', 'Teatro Goldoni'.

We were feeling our way over money and the cost of eating out, and decided on the modest tourist menu on offer in a small restaurant near the Rialto.

'It should be a lovely holiday, Jan.'

'Yes, and you're doing remarkably well,' she answered, quietly. We both knew the risk of my control breaking down through excitement at noticing this fact, so we avoided further discussion.

Everything had gone extremely well. We'd been lucky to get a lift to Heathrow from a friend, which had reduced one major source of anxiety. The drugs had worked perfectly throughout the journey. By the time I fell into bed that night they had worn off, but I was confident that I would sleep well.

I folded one of the blankets to serve as an extra pillow to support my neck, lay down and discovered that the bed was too short. I have to be able to stretch my legs out in the night to shift the rigidity that inexorably builds up, but the wooden barrier at the end of the bed was too high for me to hoist my ankles and let my feet dangle over the edge.

The banging of boats against the quayside as the wash from larger boats slammed into them made it impossible to sleep. It reminded me of the delivery of school dinners, the huge tin containers being roughly stacked outside the kitchen door. I began to work out contingency plans for moving to another hotel and constructed an explanation to give to the proprietor after already having told him we'd be staying for five nights. I began to worry for Jan, certain that she wouldn't be getting any sleep either. Then I felt the early-morning surge of fluency and numerous ideas came to mind.

It was a Saturday night and it was possible that lots of wealthy Italians would have boats moored in Venice for weekend breaks. Maybe the noise was a weekend phenomenon. But what could I do about the shortness of the bed? I'd managed to suppress my customary tendency to find someone to blame. It was usually Jan who took the brunt of this kind of unreasonable reaction, then by morning the preposterous nature of these night thoughts would become clear and my concern would be for how good a night she'd had.

I waited until after breakfast before taking any drugs. I felt an unusual lack of embarrassment as Jan fed me; the other guests either ignored me or risked snapshot glances at my shaking and trembling figure. We took the water-bus to the Accademia. The drugs hadn't worked, but I was able to shuffle round the poorly lit paintings. Suddenly, like Popeye and his spinach, control switched on as the drug penetrated my brain. I'd got used to the tremor and stiffness and was able to sit and concentrate on each picture in turn. Now that control was restored I was distracted by numerous possibilities. For a start, I was ready to go to the loo. Plans for the rest of the day crowded into my mind and I found myself skimming through the rest of the exhibition.

Jan and I made our way to the Scuola San Rocco and stretched out in the sunshine until it opened at three o'clock. Once again, because of poor light, it was a struggle to see properly, but maybe the magic of the Tintorettos wasn't entirely lost on us.

We walked back to San Marco and made the inevitable holiday blunder of sitting down and ordering a drink – the bill was five pounds. Having ruefully paid, we walked home to the hotel by a roundabout route. The din of the previous night was not repeated and by positioning myself diagonally across the bed and leaving the blankets loose at the bottom I was able to slide my feet round the end board and stretch out to my heart's content.

Early the following morning I had a run to the Piazza San Marco, down the deserted stone canyons, my feet thwacking on the damp pavement. The mist hung like cobwebs over the narrow side-canals and, as the autumn sun slanted down, creating myriad patterns of softly muted colour, the vapour over the lagoon began to evaporate, unveiling monuments to Venice's trading grandeur. The smell of freshly baked bread finally drove me back to the hotel.

After breakfast we caught the large ferry boat to the island of Torcello and sat in Attila's seat. The new drug was working extraordinarily well and sustained me through a stop-off at Burano with its miniature canal system and its souvenir shops crammed with lace and glass.

Back in the hotel I had a late-afternoon sleep which proved disastrous. To make matters worse, we had the deadline of the set evening meal in the hotel. I woke at six and took my drugs, but five minutes after we were due in the restaurant I was still lying on the bed shuddering and shaking out of control. I was filled with a mixture of sadness and anger by Jan's poorly concealed signs of irritation at my having mistimed things. The drugs finally 'took' and we were just in time. Jan wasn't too pleased when I risked ordering spaghetti, but I stayed in control and we went for our evening walk, happy that problems over my illness were surmountable.

It was still pitch dark when I woke. Quietly opening the window and shutters, from my high look-out I could see the splashes of light reflected on the water from numerous lamps, some fixed, others swinging gently in the breeze. It took about forty minutes to get ready for my run. It would be pointless going down before the proprietor had unlocked the door. He wasn't exactly friendly with his 'Good morning', but what could I expect from someone working an eighteen-hour day?

The air was cold. I felt exhilarated and alternately dashed and strolled, my arms swinging like windmills. Chugging up the arch of a bridge, tilting over the top and lightly dancing down the other side: for the next half hour, Venice was mine! This time of fluency before taking my morning dose is very precious. I longed for someone to share it with. I would have liked to buy a paper from the kiosk that was just opening but I couldn't carry it. One more goal assigned to the breaker's yard.

Back at the hotel, I stopped my feet from stomping up the stairs and quietly entered my room. It took nearly an hour to dress, manoeuvring the tremor round my limbs or locking it up in rigidity while my fingers usurped control for the delicate task of pulling on my socks. My damp T-shirt finally gave up its leech-like suction on the skin of my back, and I washed clumsily but as quickly as possible. Catching my muscles unawares, I succeeded in pouring and drinking a glass of pear juice. With my usual sadness, the drugs were swallowed. I gained full control as Jan completed the task of feeding me breakfast, then we set out on the day's programme.

On the strength of the success of the new drug so far, I had given in to the temptation to experiment with the amount I took. Whether because of this or because of a change in the weather from sunny and warm to wet and cold, the consequences were dreadful and I remained stuck in my chair. Three-quarters of an hour later we decided to set off regardless and I stumbled along while Jan did her best not to be upset.

Determined not to make allowances for the illness, I ordered a huge pizza for lunch. As Jan struggled to cut through its hard base, I tried to image some of the paintings that I had been forced to sit in front of a short time ago. I was surprised at what I could recall. The symptoms of Parkinson's had not distracted me completely. As Jan skilfully presented the last piece of pizza to my lips, I shamefacedly told her that control had just been restored.

We visited San Marco and the Doges' Palace in the rain. The rotten weather persisted throughout the evening and we decided to go on a sightseeing trip by water-bus. There was one at the landing-stage and we made a dash for it, but the effort and excitement of rushing to catch it proved too much for me and I shuddered to a halt as the controlling juice in my body petered out. We changed our plans and flopped down in a nearby restaurant out of the sheeting rain. I felt too hot, so I asked Jan to help me off with my pullover. The restaurant owner and his family looked on in horror at a man, clearly racked by cold and shivering and shaking, having his pullover removed.

'Non ha freddo?' the wife exclaimed. It was one of those occasions when I wished I could distribute printed cards containing a brief explanation of my illness and its symptoms. Jan patiently fed me my meal and, perversely, as we got up to leave control was restored.

On Wednesday morning we went to the Lido. We clambered over a hedge to reach the beach wedged between the private hotels. The uninviting water reflected the greyness of the sky and it was hard to imagine this deserted stretch of sand being overrun with crowds of sun-loving holidaymakers. We clambered back on to the road in the shadow of the lifeless casino and explored the peaceful strip of interior. Sensing the wealth behind the ornate dwellings bordering the canals, we shared vicariously in the affluence as we ordered coffee and delicious cakes at an expensive delicatessen.

Back in Venice that afternoon I got stuck in a café near the Rialto. Absurdly, I started to worry whether I was costing the owners money by overstaying. There were plenty of free seats all around and yet in my state of disability my mind was pressured to manufacture thoughts to match my miserable condition. I urged Jan to go for a look round the market and come back for me later.

Determined not to let the holiday fizzle out with a series of interrupted and cancelled projects, I shovelled down a large amount of drugs. They gave me control, but at a heavy cost in writhing movements. We spent a very enjoyable couple of hours strolling into areas not yet visited, eventually ending up back at the Piazza San Marco. We'd saved two pieces of delicious cheesecake as a treat. Having taken a single bite from my piece, my fingers, as if in spasm, flipped the rest on to the wet flagstones.

On our last day we were delighted with the Scuola San Giorgio and its display of Carpaccio's paintings, which were beautifully lit and at a height that didn't cause my neck to ache. We went for a final tour of the Grand Canal and, with our luggage on our knees at the bus station, talked happily about how everything had gone so well.

In a confident mood, I took it for granted that the municipal bus, at half the cost of the special airport service, would be perfectly adequate. It was rush-hour and in the jostling crowd I soon found myself separated from Jan. Gripping my luggage tightly with my ankles and struggling to keep hold of the metal hand-rail, I began to feel the strain of being pitched, squeezed and pushed at each of the many stops.

Two young girls had noticed my writhing head and the strained expression that had frozen on my face. At first they looked away and smiled at each other; then they started staring and finally burst out in fits of giggles. Strain turned to distress and a violent tremor spread over my whole body. They forced their gaze down and laughed out loud at my tap-dancing feet. We were nowhere near the airport and I earnestly hoped they'd be getting off soon.

We still had a long way to go and, so great was the strain that, when a man offered me his seat, I found I was crying.

At the airport I used all my tactics for keeping calm as I felt myself slipping in and out of control. Finally the agony of the queue was over and I squeezed myself into my seat. The jets began their take-off scream and we catapulted forward. Suddenly there was a hard rattling as the engines were reversed and we came to a halt halfway down the runway. I was jangling like a puppet. Jan reached over and held my hand until the plane lifted off on the third attempt. The lights of Venice disappeared from view.

Dreaming

I started writing about dreaming when Jon Alpert and I worked together on the account of Parkinson's disease. I wrote that I seem to have different phases of dreaming throughout the night. If I take medication before going to bed, which is something I rarely do, I dream profusely and the dreams are likely to have one or more of the following attributes: lucidity, by which I mean they are highly rational, logical and free of symbolism; favourability, whereby the progress and outcome of the content of the dream is likely to be attractively beneficial to my welfare; sexuality, in which the sexual element is likely to be present in the theme.

These attributes of dreaming arise provided that the amount of medication is high. What is interesting is that such qualities occur regularly around half past four in the morning. It may happen that I am having an unfavourable dream, wake up and remember it. If I go back to sleep and receive this early-morning boost, then the same dream content may be repeated, but with a much more favourable tone and outcome.

On one side of the release of transmitter all is black, or at least unfavourable. When the transmitter is released it all changes to success, an occasion for joy, triumph over others or at least a favourable outcome.

While I am dreaming, part of my dreaming may be monitoring the dream and wondering which way the outcome is going to go. I feel I am at risk and that I may get caught or may get away with it. The scarcity or abundance of resources determines the particular treatment given to whatever theme is developed for a dream.

The most interesting dreams are those that span the boost of transmitter. This produces ongoing revisions to the slant, colour or outcome of the dream. If I wake, experience the increased muscular fluency of the morning boost and go back to sleep instead of going for a run, the dream that had been progressing unfavourably is converted to success, rationality and a flooding of sexual arousal.

I peer down the drive. My car is missing. After some moments' reflection about where I left it, I accept the fact that it's been stolen. A few moments later I look down the drive again and see a crumpled, crushed car sticking out of a neighbour's driveway. Is it mine? I take a close look and refocus on the drive of another neighbour. I find my car undamaged. I wake with an erection!

However, if I stay asleep long after the boost and don't get up until, say, eight o'clock, I am likely to be in a worse state in respect of muscular fluency than if I'd got up early, gone for a three-mile run, returned and organised my own breakfast – activities which one might expect to be very expensive in terms of resources.

This heavy depletion of resources is often reflected in the content of the dream if I sleep in late, where there is a change from favourable to unfavourable.

I'm walking up a wide staircase in a grand house. I'm holding on to a rail and chatting animatedly with Paul McCartney. We enter a large room, walk over to the window and pass through to a balcony where we sip drinks and take in the warmth of the strong sunlight. Later I try to descend the stairs, but find them blocked by a huge pillar. There is only a narrow passage with no rail for support. I look over the edge and get a feeling of vertigo. I don't dare to pass. I turn back, enter a classroom and self-consciously pick my way to the back, where I worry that the other children will be angry with me for disturbing their lesson.

I wake up. My legs feel stiff and I am in far worse a state than before I fell asleep.

I'd discussed dreaming with Jonathan Miller.

'When you dream, how often do you dream of yourself unimpeded by the tremor or rigidity? Do you see yourself as healthy in your dreams?'

'I frequently dream in a way whereby the deficit doesn't enter the situation, where I'm completely free of the deficit. If I'm asleep and the deficit manifests itself, I might dream about the deficit.'

'You mean you dream about yourself with tremor?'

'I can't be clear on this. I do occasionally dream of myself in a state of tremor with an audience reacting in one way or another.'

'Unfavourably?'

'I can't say. When I'm low on the drug, the content of the dream provided by the previous day's unfinished business and concerns is cast in an unfavourable light. If the level of transmitter is high, I dream the content in such a way that I am successful. In other words, if there is plenty of transmitter, I win. If I'm low, I lose.

'Perhaps a better way to account for the occasions when the deficit crops up in my dreams is to distinguish between the roles of participant and spectator. When I simply participate, things may go well for me and there's no experience of Parkinsonian symptoms. On the other hand, I may have trouble. This either reflects or is reflected in slowness so that I miss deadlines, and in loss of postural control resulting in me struggling along on all fours. Tremor seems not to arise then, perhaps linked to the fact that it fades away during sleep.

'Now if resources are sufficiently high I may adopt the role of spectator. Then, instead of having a dream experience of Parkinson's, I'm observing this person – me – and noticing the fact that he – I – have difficulty moving, gets stuck and even has tremor.'

'How much of a dreamer were you before you became ill?'

'I suspect I stopped dreaming to a tremendous extent during the years leading up to the time when Parkinson's manifested itself and it is only since taking the drugs that dreaming has been re-established.'

'Are your dreams vivid, colourful and active now?'

'Very. They range from those where I lose, miss trains, overshoot deadlines, get mugged – and once I dreamt I died – to the other end of the scale where I win, am successful, triumphant, surmount all difficulties, reason my way through complex problems and so on.'

'In the dreams of failure, are you afflicted by tremor or rigidity, or are they dreams of failure for other reasons?'

'That's interesting. There is a link, of course. Is my failure to catch the train because I'm slow merely an ordinary failure, or is it an expression of the slowness of movement that is a symptom of Parkinsonism? Does my failure to accomplish a task reflect the Parkinson patient's difficulty in co-ordinating actions and planning complex manoeuvres?'

'Do you ever visualise yourself being frustrated by tremor or rigidity or slowness of movement?'

'Rarely. In fact, I can't remember a single instance.'

'So there is no immediate subjective representation of Parkinsonism in the dreamwork?'

'No. It suggests that my self-image as a person without Parkinson's wins out during the night.'

'So that it is about success or failure regardless of Parkinsonism?'

'I suspect that the impact on my psyche of the times when I'm in full control has a much greater impact than moments when I'm out of control.'

'How many of the dreams are specifically physical in nature and how many are social or intellectual?'

'I can't say. All three kinds of theme feature in my dreams. In a debate at college I might win or lose in advancing my arguments. Running for a train, I may catch it or miss it. If I've taken a lot of drugs, I wake up with solutions to complex problems that have been exercising me the previous day.

'The drugs are matched directly with what is lacking in my brain. They provide the means for fluent movement, memory, thought and creativity. Dreaming draws on all of these, and the level of transmitter leaves its stamp on the flavour or favourability with which the subconscious treats the content of the dream.'

A Dinner Party

'Of all the aids for my illness, the best by far is the straw. Besides drinks, it's good for yoghurt, custard and even porridge. As long as you're willing to put up with the noise, it allows you to get to those favourite last bits,' I told our dinner-party guests as I handed round drinks.

We all drifted into the dining room and sat down at the table. John was the first to notice.

'Do I see something that I've got to try to ignore?'

'I went to the occupational-therapy place and they gave me these to try.'

'Carry on, Ive,' said Phil. 'We'll try not to look.'

'I'm going to look. I think they're cute,' said Gillie.

I was in a very good state for the meal. I had taken drugs earlier in the day, had a sleep in the late afternoon and was now enjoying the benefits of storage. There was quite a bit of tremor, but I could shift it around to feed myself for most of the meal. The main thing was that I was able to join in the spirit of the occasion and not have to sit quietly, perhaps with muscular control but thoroughly dampened and disinclined to join in.

I pulled out a couple more exhibits and began using the one that John had been quick to spot. It was a short, stubby fork with a bulky handle of foam-rubber. It was useless. As I took hold of it, my fingers could not get a grip and what little food I succeeded in picking up was quickly shaken off, back on to the plate.

'Let's try the spoon!'

The round scoop came out at right-angles from the handle. Presumably it was for someone with arthritis who could not move his wrist. I found it difficult to line it up with my mouth. It might be useful if you wanted to feed over your shoulder without taking the baby out of its harness. The last two implements were a fork and spoon, both eighteen inches long with fat foam handles. The idea was that you put your elbows on the table and levered the food to your mouth as if with a dockyard crane. As I began to demonstrate eating the soup with croûtons, the guests near me edged away in nervous anticipation.

'I'll come and feed you, Ive,' said Ellen.

'Thanks, but I'm OK for the moment. I'll use my straw and scoop up the croûtons at the end.'

'OK, but you know I like feeding you. I really do.'

'Oh well, perhaps the old sex appeal's not dead after all!' I thought.

How difficult it must be to design equipment to help disabled people and how inappropriate for me most of it seemed to be. My top three 'aids' would be a straw, a bidet and a walk-in shower, in that order!

Epilogue

Why is it so important to me to manage my drug-taking and not just take drugs every couple of hours or according to a simple routine established by my doctor? Apart from the main reason of wanting to retain personal control, there is a functional advantage in managing on an optimum minimum amount. The drugs are not a magic cure, they have side-effects, the most obvious of which is dyskinesia or writhing.

My body is possessed of two demons. Off the drugs, with too little dopamine in the system, I suffer the three classic symptoms of Parkinsonism: trembling, rigidity and slowness of movement. Sometimes this first demon takes hold of my body and tries to shake my teeth loose. At other times, the tremor can be controlled by shifting it round the body. It's hard work. I lie on my bed and am able to think clearly and analytically, but my speech is a slow, quiet monotone. I half close my eyes or focus on the twining vine painted on my bedroom wall. Movement is difficult. I stoop, hollow-chested, and shuffle along by tilting forwards and collapsing into motion.

With surplus drugs swilling around in my bloodstream, another demon takes over and my body begins to writhe to a different tune. My arms seem double-jointed as they snake up to my face, the hands bending grotesquely at right-angles. My head cocks back and to one side, nose stabbing forwards, rimless spectacles perched on the prominent bridge like a quizzical, manic secretary bird. My lips purse and blow small bubbles that make popping sounds, my eyes bulge slightly and my head twitches and bobs uncontrollably.

If control can be achieved through stored resources, then both demons are held at bay. It seems as if the drugs can be transformed by the brain into dopamine, which is then stored. These moments, minutes, hours become magical, to be treasured for the balm they provide. Above all, it creates choice. I can choose whether to dip into stored resources or not, to harbour and spin out muscular control or to blow it in a spurt of action. When the drugs are operating via the bloodstream, I am pushed into activity with little or no opportunity to intervene.

The best state to be in is after the drugs take but before my writhing demon gains control. Lying on my bed waiting for the drugs to take, I suddenly notice the creak of my leather trainers as I stretch when the drugs 'take'. I curl my feet, lift my hands together over my head and stretch my whole body like a cat until I can lie straight.

Of the two demons, I prefer the drugless rather than the drugged. In other words, I prefer the moderately 'off' state in which I am coping by drawing on stored resources. Yet there can be massive pressure from doctors (who should know better) and people around me to take as many drugs as are necessary to mask the symptoms of Parkinson's – but these people do not fully admit the consequences and discomfort of L-dopa's side-effects. You can manage more easily on the drugs; you are less of a burden on those around you; but the social consequences of the writhing side-effects can be as daunting to the sufferer as the symptoms they 'cure'.

This idea of storage, of being able to cope by drawing on resources processed and stored, may simply be a huge rationalisation, an excuse for my developing a unique way of taking the drugs which allows me to retain control. But I don't think so. These magic moments are the only times when I am whole again and unpossessed.

This book is very much my personal account of myself and my illness. The decision to write it created a dilemma for Jan. She said she would have preferred me not to do it at all, as she wanted to live her life privately and resented the public exposure involved in television programmes or autobiographies. Nevertheless, she read through the manuscript and made a number of very helpful suggestions. Some things, however, she saw from an entirely different perspective. I suggested she might like to add footnotes or write a postscript to give her the opportunity to correct what she saw as any false impressions, but she felt she wouldn't be able to put her side of the story adequately in that way and, anyway, she didn't want to write about herself.

She also objected to the black-and-white way in which I had presented our early disagreements over the drugs, and felt that I had oversimplified her attitude. Certainly there was a philosophical issue about taking drugs, but that ignored the stark choice we'd been faced with: either I took the drugs or I became immobile and helpless.

As there was nothing she could do to stop me writing the book, and because she wouldn't try to do so even if she could, Jan wanted to be left out of it. But people had made inferences when she had been omitted from the television programme. 'Oh that poor man, struggling to feed himself. What sort of a wife must he have!' Protestations that there had been a television crew of nine watching my struggles didn't seem to alleviate the criticism.

In truth, I couldn't hope to have a more sustaining companion. I wanted her to support my desire to be self-determining and independent. What an impossible paradox! And what an uncomfortable role for Jan. Despite everything, she generously said, as on so many other occasions, that she would put her personal quandaries aside and stand by me in what I wanted to do.

At a dinner party to celebrate finishing the book, Steve asked what I would do next.

'An opera,' I said.

'On ice!' added Jan.

The author would be pleased to hear about the ideas and experiences of anyone with an interest in Parkinson's disease. His address is

> 26 Panton Street
> Cambridge
> CB2 1HP

A copy of the *Listener* article may be obtained by sending a medium-sized SAE to the above address.

If you wish to make use of the Parkinson's Disease Society, the address is

> 39 Portland Place
> London
> W1N 3DG

A monthly newsletter summarising the most recent medical, social and psychological aspects of Parkinson's disease is available from Ivan Vaughan at the above address, for residents of the UK; or from

> Parkinson's Disease Update
> Medical Publishing Company
> P.O. Box 24622
> Philadelphia
> PA 19111
> USA